NATURAL MENOPAUSE REMEDIES

Which Drug-Free Cures *Really* Work

**Other books authored or coauthored by
Nadine Taylor, M.S., R.D.**

Green Tea

If You Think You Have an Eating Disorder

Arthritis for Dummies

25 Natural Ways to Relieve PMS

What Your Doctor May Not Tell You About

Hypertension

NATURAL MENOPAUSE REMEDIES

Which Drug-Free Cures *Really* Work

Nadine Taylor, M.S., R.D.

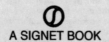

A SIGNET BOOK

SIGNET
Published by New American Library, a division of
Penguin Group (USA) Inc., 375 Hudson Street,
New York, New York 10014, U.S.A.
Penguin Books Ltd, 80 Strand,
London WC2R 0RL, England
Penguin Books Australia Ltd, 250 Camberwell Road,
Camberwell, Victoria 3124, Australia
Penguin Books Canada Ltd, 10 Alcorn Avenue,
Toronto, Ontario, Canada M4V 3B2
Penguin Books (N.Z.) Ltd, Cnr Rosedale and Airborne Roads,
Albany, Auckland 1310, New Zealand

Penguin Books Ltd, Registered Offices:
80 Strand, London WC2R 0RL, England

First published by Signet, an imprint of New American Library,
a division of Penguin Group (USA) Inc.

First Printing, January 2004
10 9 8 7 6 5 4 3 2 1

 REGISTERED TRADEMARK—MARCA REGISTRADA

Printed in the United States of America

PUBLISHER'S NOTE
Every effort has been made to ensure that the information contained in this
book is complete and accurate. However, neither the publisher nor the author is engaged in rendering professional advice or services to the individual
reader. The ideas, procedures, and suggestions contained in this book are
not intended as a substitute for consulting with your physician. All matters
regarding your health require medical supervision. Neither the author nor
the publisher shall be liable or responsible for any loss or damage allegedly
arising from any information or suggestion in this book.

For Dawn—It's been rough sailing,
but the future is bright!

Contents

Chapter One

You're 45? Here, Take These Hormones!

Like just about every other woman my age (40-plus), I am approaching menopause with a mixture of elation and dread. The elation springs from the thought of no more periods and no more fear of getting pregnant (hooray!). The dread comes in when I think of my bones turning to honeycomb, regular meltdowns due to hot flashes, my skin wrinkling and sagging, and my reproductive organs shrinking and shriveling. Yes, when I weigh the advantages of menopause against the disadvantages, there's really no contest: I'd much rather deal with the messiness of periods and the risk of unplanned pregnancy than with the loss of my trusty female hormones.

But frankly, up until about a year ago I wasn't worrying too much about hormone loss and its accompanying long-term effects, because (a) I wasn't experiencing much discomfort on the menopausal front, and (b) I knew that if I did, I could always fall back on hormone replacement therapy (HRT). And why wouldn't I have faith in HRT? The medical profession, the media, and my college health textbooks all concurred: HRT was the way to go if you wanted to ward off heart disease, protect your bones, fight colon cancer, and otherwise avoid turning into the Little Old Lady from Pasadena.

Although it was touted as a modern day "fountain of youth" (or at least a "fountain of holding the line"), HRT did come with a few drawbacks. There was a slightly increased risk of breast cancer, and there was a chance of developing uterine cancer if you took estrogen without progesterone. But for most women the benefits of HRT outweighed the risks—or so the experts told us. By the 1980s it seemed like everybody past a certain age, including my own mother, was taking hormones. In fact, it became almost de rigueur for doctors to prescribe female hormones to just about any woman past the age of 45, *whether or not she had any symptoms of menopause.* As a result, millions of women were gobbling synthetic hormone pills on a daily basis—often, without knowing why.

The "Miracle Cure" for Menopause

Hormone replacement therapy was conceived back in the late 1950s, during our country's love affair with chemicals. It began simply as estrogen replacement therapy (ERT), and was designed to combat hot flashes, ease psychological problems, and keep women "forever young" (male-doctor-speak for "interested in sex—and not too dried out to enjoy it"). Throughout the 1960s, estrogen became more and more popular, until someone finally noticed that a great many of the women taking it were developing cancer of the lining of the uterus (endometrial cancer). Sure enough, the cause of the cancer was eventually traced to the use of ERT. So the idea of taking hormones lost popularity for a few years, until it was proven that taking progesterone or progestins (synthetic forms of progesterone) along with estrogen could negate the cancer risk, while preserving the "miracle cure" aspects of the therapy. The estrogen-progesterone combo was referred to as "hormone replacement therapy," or HRT. Thus, ERT was replaced by HRT.

Thanks to the relentless marketing campaigns of the big drug companies and to media hungry for sensational medical "breakthroughs," it didn't take long until the whole country piled onto the HRT bandwagon. Doctors and their female patients alike rushed to embrace the pill that would not only preserve youth but prevent two of the most dreaded diseases of old age: heart disease and osteoporosis. This attitude fit right in with our hormone-popping culture, in which some girls started taking birth control pills as early as age 13. Often, women who had been on the pill for a decade or more continued taking it right up until they were hit with the symptoms of impending menopause, and even then they might go on taking it. In 1998, my own gynecologist told me that she often prescribed birth control pills to help ease symptoms of hormonal fluctuations in her patients in perimenopause (the four-year period beginning two years before the final menstrual period). Then, once these women had eased into menopause, she'd switch them to hormone replacement therapy. So it was completely possible for a woman to start taking hormones as a teenager and continue right up until she died of old age. Yet no one has ever measured the long-term effects of this decades-long barrage of hormones on the female body.[1]

It Sounds Good to Me. . . .

I started experimenting with hormones at the tender age of 19, taking birth control pills off and on for about the next ten years before giving them up for good. I got major yeast infections, and I was tired of swallowing chemicals every day, especially during the times I wasn't sexually active. A diaphragm seemed less invasive.

In my thirties I went back to college to study nutrition and become a Registered Dietitian. Immersed in the study of physiology, health, nutrition, and medicines, I was exposed to a certain amount of research on hormone replacement therapy, and my professors repeated the standard beliefs of the day. Estrogen combined with progesterone is very beneficial to the health of most women, they said. It protects against heart disease and osteoporosis and possibly colon cancer. It won't cause uterine cancer (as long as you keep taking your progesterone), and the risk of breast cancer is slight. It also keeps your skin smooth, your breasts from sagging, your vagina moist, and so forth. I was sold. I decided then and there that I was definitely going to take HRT when my time came.

In my forties, out of the blue, I became a raging insomniac (or an insomniac who felt like raging due to the chronic lack of sleep). When I finally did drop off, my sleep was light and fitful. My doctor pronounced me perimenopausal and gave me a prescription for HRT, even though I was still getting my regular periods. I started taking the drug. Unfortunately, my sleeplessness continued, and suddenly I had a few more problems to go along with it: bloating, weight gain, and anxiety. I chalked it up to the "change of life."

Then one day I was talking to a naturopathic physician, who said: "Why are you taking estrogen when you're still getting your period? If you've got a period, you've obviously got enough estrogen already. Getting too much could be the cause of your symptoms."

Why *was* I taking estrogen, anyway? Here I was, with a master's degree in one of the health professions, and I was just as naïve about hormone replacement as anybody else. My doctor had said, "Take these pills," and I had nodded and gobbled them up. I stopped taking HRT then and there and started reading up on the subject of menopause and perimenopause. I learned about natural progesterone and how it could help correct hormone imbalances, especially during the perimenopause stage. I got rid of the synthetic hormones and substituted some natural progesterone, and my sleep problem gradually disappeared.

The HERS Study

Believe it or not, although women had been taking HRT for decades to ward off heart disease, no one really knew if it worked. For years, studies had shown that HRT had a positive effect on certain *indicators* of heart disease, like blood cholesterol, atherosclerosis, and blood pressure. It appeared that taking HRT could decrease the kinds of cholesterol that clogged your arteries and increase the kinds that cleaned your arteries out. Although this doesn't necessarily mean that those taking HRT *would* end up having fewer heart attacks or strokes, scientists figured that this would probably be the case. So, in a sense, we were all guinea pigs, taking our hormones strictly on faith.

The Difference Between Natural and Synthetic Hormones

Natural hormones are substances that are identical to those produced in your body. Synthetic hormones are enough like the natural kind to get into the cell and perform some of the same functions, but they don't provide all of the benefits. And they do have some definite detriments.

For example, both natural progesterone and its synthetic counterparts (the progestins) help prevent uterine cancer. But only natural progesterone helps to protect against breast cancer, normalize the fatty acid profile, restore normal sex drive, and regulate sleep patterns. Progestins, on the other hand, contribute to mood swings, fatigue, depression, insomnia, bloating, breast tenderness, weight gain, and anxiety—none of which are side effects of natural progesterone use.

Synthetic estrogens are altered in the laboratory so that drug companies can patent them (think Premarin). They tend to be stronger and more toxic than estrogens manufactured naturally in the human body; thus they increase your odds of suffering from symptoms of estrogen dominance (weight gain, bloating, anxiety, depression, low blood sugar) and from estrogen-related diseases (breast and uterine cancer). The natural forms of estrogen (estradiol, estrone, and estriol) tend to be safer.

It's important to note that *most studies of hormone replacement therapy involve the use of synthetic hormones.* Don't automatically assume that *all* hormone replacement therapy brings about the same scary results we've seen in the recent studies, all of which used synthetic hormones. We're in dire need of some good long-term studies on the effects of natural HRT to distinguish between the effects of the natural and synthetic versions of both progesterone and estrogen.

Then, in 1994, researchers set up the Heart and Estrogen/Progestin Replacement Study (HERS),[2] which was designed to see how hormone replacement therapy would affect women who already had heart disease. They gathered together 2,763 women who were postmenopausal, still had their uteruses (they hadn't had hysterectomies), and already had heart disease. The women were randomly divided into two groups; during a four-year period, those in one group were given a daily dose of HRT (the equivalent of one PREMPRO tablet),[3] those in the other group, a placebo. The results were surprising. The hormone group *didn't fare any better* than the placebo group as far as heart disease was concerned: 172 women in the hormone group versus 176 women in the placebo group had either had a heart attack or died due to coronary heart disease by the study's end. The hormones only "saved" four women, and there were some definite negative aspects. During the first year of the study, the hormone users were three times more likely to develop blood clots and 52 percent more likely to have heart attacks than those given the placebo. During subsequent years, however, these risks did subside to equal those of the placebo group.

Still, the meaning was clear: Using a combination of estrogen and progestin did not reduce the risk of heart attack or death due to coronary disease. In fact, women who already had heart disease and who took these hormones were slightly *more* likely to have a heart attack, at least during the first couple years of therapy.

Strike one against HRT.

The ERA Study

Some of the same researchers who worked on the HERS study later moved on to the Estrogen Replacement and Atherosclerosis trial,[4] nicknamed ERA, the results of which were published in the *New England Journal of Medicine* in 2000. The idea was to see if women whose coronary arteries were clogged would be able to decrease the clogging through the use of HRT.

For the ERA trial, 309 women with at least one narrowed coronary artery were assigned randomly to one of three groups: the estrogen group, the estrogen-plus-progestin group, or the placebo group. Each woman took one pill daily (without knowing what she was getting). The women in the group were followed for an average of 3.2 years. The result: The narrowing of the blood vessels of the women in each of the three groups remained virtually the same. In other words, the hormones did nothing to control the buildup of plaque inside the heart's arteries, which is a major risk factor for heart attacks and stroke.

Strike two against HRT.

The Women's Health Initiative
Clinical Trial

Then came the biggest study of them all—the Women's Health Initiative,[5] called WHI for short.

Backed by the National Institutes of Health, this was the one everybody had been waiting for. It was the first large-scale, long-term, randomized, placebo-controlled, double blind study of the effects of HRT on several important areas, including the brain, the bones, and the heart, and the incidence of cancer in more than 16,000 women.

Postmenopausal women between the ages of 50 and 79 who had intact uteruses were recruited at forty clinical centers around the country. As in the HERS study, they were randomly assigned to one of two groups: those taking PREMPRO, and those taking a placebo. The women were supposed to be followed for an average of 8.5 years, with the study set to conclude in March 2005.

But with almost three years to go before the end of the study, a bomb dropped. The National Institutes of Health decided to pull the plug on the WHI study because it was clear that the women taking the hormones were at an *increased risk for breast cancer, blood clots, heart attacks, and strokes.* Although the increases in risk were small, they were statistically significant. Researchers estimated that for every 10,000 women taking HRT, there would be 8 extra cases of breast cancer or stroke, 7 extra cases of heart attack, and 18 extra cases of blood clots. The good news was that there would be an average of 5 fewer cases of hip fracture and 6 fewer cases of colon cancer. But the health risks outweighed the benefits, and the researchers felt it was unethical to expose their subjects to any more danger.

The news was stunning: Not only did HRT fail to protect women against heart attacks, strokes, and dangerous blood clots, it actually *increased* the odds that they would suffer from them. Add to that an amplified risk of breast cancer, and you've got some pretty good reasons to stay away from hormone replacement therapy.

Strike three against HRT.

So Now What?

The bad news about HRT has left women and health professionals reeling. We might have expected the increase in breast cancer, since estrogen is like fertilizer for that kind of cancer. But no one imagined that HRT would make us even more likely to develop heart disease. Suddenly, doctors across the nation are telling their menopausal patients to get off of HRT immediately. "There are plenty of other drugs you can take to ward off heart disease or osteoporosis," they'll tell you, as they dash off a handful of new prescriptions. But for those of us who feel that we've already taken more than enough drugs, this approach may not be too appealing.

So it's only natural to turn to the "natural" or alternative therapies. And they're out there in droves. Just about everywhere you turn, somebody's touting yet another natural approach to curing menopausal troubles: dong quai, soy, red clover, vitamin E, acupuncture, herbs. The list goes on and on. But which of these, if any, have actual proof that they work? For many of these alternatives, there's plenty of hype but very little scientific backup. And what about side effects? Haven't we just learned from the HRT fiasco that the side effects of an otherwise good cure can render the whole thing useless?

What You'll Find in This Book

In an attempt to answer these questions and more, I plunged into the scientific literature and organized what I found into book form. I've arranged it according to the most common menopausal problems and symptoms, such as heart disease, osteoporosis, hot flashes, and vaginal changes. Chapters 4 through 12 are divided into two main sections: "The Problem" and "What You Can Do About It." In "The Problem," I discuss a major menopausal symptom or problem, what causes it, and who's most likely to suffer from it. In the "What You Can Do About It" section, I explain in detail the scientifically proven ways of easing the problem or symptom, divided into the categories of general diet, specific foods and phytochemicals, vitamins and minerals, exercise, and, where applicable, lifestyle changes. For each cure, I include the typical dosage and method of administration, and any cautions or contraindications. At the end of most chapters is a short section called "Rising Stars" highlighting some promising newcomers that with further study may prove to be helpful.

But before immersing ourselves in symptoms and cures, let's take a brief look at the nuts and bolts of the female reproductive system, the phenomenon of menopause, and the ways in which hormone replacement therapy affects the body.

Chapter Two

What Is This Thing Called Menopause?

The word "menopause" comes from the Latin words *mensis* (month) and *pausa* (end) and refers to the end of the monthly menstrual period. Simply put, menopause is the permanent shutting down of your baby-making factory. It's part of a process called the *climacteric*, which involves the fluctuation and gradual decline of the production of female hormones, starting (believe it or not) when you're in your late twenties or early thirties. The process continues over a period of thirty-five years or longer, until your hormones finally settle down to low but steady levels in your late fifties or early sixties.

This hormonal decline is so subtle that at first you probably won't notice anything. But somewhere along the way, usually between the ages of 35 and 45, your hormone levels and your menstrual cycles will start to fluctuate. Your periods will become irregular and will sometimes be lighter or heavier than usual. You can find yourself irritable, depressed, and prone to headaches. Sleep may elude you and you may gain weight. Fatigue, low sexual desire, and water retention may also plague you. It feels like a bad case of premenstrual syndome (PMS), but it's actually *perimenopause*, a period of wildly fluctuating hormone levels that begins about two years before your final menstrual period and continues for approximately two more years. The cause of these miserable symptoms: chemical imbalances due to the drop in production of the hormones estrogen and progesterone. Perimenopause overlaps with *menopause*, the point in time when your ovaries stop releasing eggs and menstruation ends for good. So, technically, you can be perimenopausal and postmenopausal at the same time. *Premenopause* is the period when you're on the verge of menopause but you haven't experienced any typical menopausal symptoms, like hot flashes or vaginal dryness. Your periods may be starting to become irregular, but that's about it.

Menopause, the Event

Contrary to what most people think, menopause is not a process but a single event. It officially occurs the day after your final menstrual period ends, but you won't know for sure that it's happened until another 12 months have passed. At that point you can backtrack a year to the end of your last period and you'll know when this important event took place.

The average North American woman enters menopause at about age 50, but menopause may occur as early as age 40 or as late as age 55. In general, about 85 percent of women will have entered menopause by age 52. While race, socioeconomic status, marital status, and geographical location don't seem to influence the age that it begins, menopause can be brought on prematurely by smoking, autoimmune disorders that damage the ovaries, and genetic predisposition. Surgery to remove the ovaries or cut back on their blood supply, radiation to the pelvis, or chemotherapy can induce *artificial menopause*, and this will cause the same symptoms as natural menopause. A hysterectomy (surgical removal of the uterus) will cause menstrual periods to stop, but it won't induce menopause because the ovaries will continue to function.

But before we take a look at how the gradual shutting down of the reproductive system can affect us, let's remind ourselves of how things worked when the system was humming along at its peak.

The "Philhormonic Symphony"

Complex chemical substances called *hormones* regulate the activity of the reproductive organs. You can think of the hormones and the glands that produce them as something akin to a small orchestra. Each member of the orchestra performs certain highly specialized functions and provides its own beautiful music. They are

- *the corpus luteum*—the part of the follicle that's left behind by the egg after ovulation; it secretes progesterone during the second half of the menstrual cycle
- *estradiol*—a potent form of estrogen that stimulates the release of FSH and LH, causing ovulation
- *estrogen*—a hormone that prepares the uterus for

the fertilization, implantation, and nutritional support of an embryo
- *the follicle*—a coating that protects the egg while it grows and matures and that also produces estrogen
- *follicle-stimulating hormone (FSH)*—a hormone that stimulates the growth and maturation of an egg
- *luteinizing hormone (LH)*—a hormone that causes ovulation and stimulates the production of progesterone
- *the pituitary gland*—a small gland located at the base of the brain that stimulates the release of numerous hormones that govern the reproductive cycle
- *progesterone*—a hormone that prepares the uterus for reception of a fertilized egg

When all elements of this "reproductive orchestra" are in peak form and playing properly, they will blend together and create a wonderful harmony. Their highest purpose, of course, is the creation of a new life. But the harmony of their "music" also positively affects the entire body—the brain, the bones, the cardiovascular system, the skin—and even the emotions. The music created by the female reproductive system is like a movement in a symphony, one that lasts between 26 and 28 days. In general, it starts out quietly, reaches a crescendo at midpoint in the cycle, then drifts back down to near silence toward the end.

The Music Begins

The movement begins on Day 1, the first day of menstruation. Sometime during the first few days of the cycle, the hypothalamus (a sort of control center in the brain) sends a signal to the *pituitary gland,* saying, "Let's get some eggs ready for fertilization. Start the music."

The pituitary responds by producing *follicle-stimulating hormone* (FSH) and *luteinizing hormone* (LH). FSH sounds a trumpet call, triggering the production of *estrogen* and the growth of anywhere from three to thirty of the eggs residing in the ovaries. Each of these eggs is encased in a protective coating called a *follicle,* a neat little wrapper that doubles as a hormone factory. As the eggs increase in size, the follicles also grow, and soon they, too, begin to produce estrogen.

Estrogen is the dominant hormone of the first half of the menstrual cycle. It thickens the lining of the uterus and makes the blood vessels in the uterine wall start to grow. Then, if a fertilized egg should suddenly appear, it will have a nice, nutrient-rich place in which to lodge. As the follicles grow larger during the first two weeks of the cycle, they produce more and more estrogen, causing the estrogen music to rise in pitch and volume. Finally, one of the follicles emerges as the largest and best developed of all and, like a queen bee, becomes the one to provide this month's egg.

During these first two weeks, the music of LH is soft, although it is building gradually. Then, around Day 13 of the cycle, when estrogen levels climax in a blast of their most potent form, *estradiol,* both LH and FSH levels surge upward. They hit their own climaxes on Day 14, causing the ripened egg to burst through its follicle (a process called *ovulation*). Free at last, the egg is launched on a journey through the fallopian tube toward the uterus in search of viable sperm. And that's just the first half of the story.

The Symphony Continues

During the second part of the cycle, things change and new melodies are heard. The trusty old follicle, which has now been discarded by the egg, suddenly transforms itself into a potent hormone factory and takes on a new identity as the *corpus luteum*. It continues to produce estrogen but adds a brand-new offering: large amounts of *progesterone*. This makes the lining of the uterus spongy and more hospitable to the fertilized egg. Progesterone becomes the dominant hormone during the second half of the cycle. As progesterone levels build toward a climax, estrogen chimes in and heads for its second peak, while FSH and LH decrease and recede into the background.

Around Day 23, estrogen and progesterone levels reach a crescendo. But if the egg hasn't been fertilized and implanted in the uterine wall by this time, the music rapidly begins to fade. The thickened lining of the uterus breaks down, and within about five days the hormonal music dwindles until it's nearly gone. The symphonic movement has concluded and the process of shedding the lining of the uterus begins Day 1 of a new menstrual cycle.

A Sour Note

But what happens when not all of the instrumental lines are played to perfection? What if somebody skips a beat, slows down, or plays badly? It's easy to see how formerly beautiful music can go sour. That's what happens when your hormone levels start to fluctuate and drop off, and striking hormonal balance becomes hit or miss. The symptoms of hormonal imbalance and decline are what we commonly refer to as "going through menopause."

A Delicate Balance: The Relationship Between Estrogen and Progesterone

Like two kids on a seesaw, estrogen and progesterone work in opposition to maintain hormonal balance. But they also help sensitize receptors for each other throughout the body. That is, progesterone helps the body take up and use estrogen, and estrogen helps the body take up and use progesterone.

Estrogen is responsible for the creation of the curvy female form. It promotes cell growth, which is why it can be dangerous in the presence of certain estrogen-dependent cancers, like those of the breast, ovaries or uterine lining. It's also responsible for increased body fat, retention of salt and fluid, and a decrease in the sex drive. All of this makes sense when the body is being prepared for motherhood.

Progesterone, on the other hand, helps keep estrogen in line. While estrogen promotes the buildup of the uterine lining, progesterone triggers the breakdown and shedding of that lining. (Estrogen is almost never prescribed without progesterone for a woman who has an intact uterus, because estrogen will cause overgrowth of the uterine lining, which can lead to cancer.) While estrogen increases body fat, progesterone helps the body use that fat for energy. Estrogen impairs the sex drive; progesterone restores it. Estrogen increases blood clotting; progesterone normalizes it. Together, these two hormones keep the female reproductive system, and many other bodily functions, working in perfect harmony.

Unfortunately, the harmony doesn't last forever. During perimenopause, when ovulation becomes sporadic, there will be some months when there's no corpus luteum produced to manufacture progesterone. During those months, your progesterone levels

are near zero—as low as those found in postmenopausal women. Yet your estrogen production will
continue as if nothing has happened. This creates a
phenomenon called *estrogen dominance*, in which estrogen is allowed to "run wild" without the balancing effect of progesterone. The unhappy result is a
long list of symptoms familiar to many women experiencing perimenopause. Weight gain, bloating,
breast tenderness, low blood sugar, fatigue, lack of
sex drive, migraine headaches, irritability, and emotional hypersensitivity are all common indications of
too much estrogen and not enough progesterone. If
this sounds like PMS, that's because PMS is often
due to estrogen dominance, as well.

Symptoms of Estrogen Excess / Progesterone Deficiency

- anxiety
- depression
- emotional hypersensitivity
- fatigue
- fibrocystic breasts
- food cravings (sweets, caffeine, carbohydrates)
- headaches
- irritability
- low blood sugar
- low sex drive
- mood swings
- sleeplessness
- sluggish metabolism
- uterine fibroids
- water retention
- weight gain

Is It PMS, Perimenopause, or the "Real Thing"?

If you've got symptoms of estrogen excess/progesterone deficiency and you're wondering how far along you are in the menopausal process, think about it this way: If you're still getting your period regularly, your symptoms are probably due to PMS. If your period has become sporadic, perimenopause may be the culprit.

As for determining whether or not you've gone through the "event" of menopause, the best way is to get your FSH (follicle-stimulating hormone) levels tested. During the reproductive years, FSH is typically below 10 mIU/ml, but it rises as menopause nears. Once FSH has exceeded 30 mIU/ml, you've probably "made the grade." Other indications that can confirm your postmenopausal status are high levels of LH (greater than 20 mIU/ml) and low levels of a potent form of estrogen called estradiol (less than 20 pg/ml).

When the Music Starts to Change: Signs and Symptoms of Menopause

Many of the symptoms of PMS or perimenopause are also symptoms of menopause, since progesterone deficiency is common to all of these conditions. But menopause has the added wallop of estrogen deficiency, bringing on additional side effects that can run the gamut from physical to mental to emotional. While some lucky women have just one symptom—loss of the menstrual period—others can suffer from several. The most common signs and symptoms of menopause include the following:

Permanent Loss of the Menstrual Cycle

During the decade or so before your menstrual periods stop completely, the number of follicles in your ovaries decreases markedly. While your ovaries contained about 400,000 follicles when you were born, by the time you're 40 you'll have less than 10,000. And, like surly teenagers, the follicles that are still hanging around won't respond too well to the promptings of FSH and LH. Your ovaries begin to produce less and less estrogen and fewer and fewer eggs. Even though your menstrual periods may continue as usual, ovulation becomes sporadic, skipping a month or two. (These are called *anovulatory cycles*.)

Eventually, your ovaries won't be able to produce enough estrogen to keep your menstrual cycle going on a monthly basis, so skipped periods, lighter periods, and longer "dry spells" between periods become common. A lack of progesterone due to anovulatory cycles can allow excessive buildup of the uterine lining, which may be followed by unusually heavy periods. Finally, estrogen levels drop to the point where the menstrual cycle shuts down completely.

Hot Flashes and Night Sweats

No one is exactly sure what causes hot flashes and night sweats. They typically begin before menopause (sometimes years before the menstrual period ends) and decline markedly once menopause occurs, although they may continue for a few months to several years past menopause. Hot flashes are common at night (and are often called "night sweats") or during stressful times. They can occur once in awhile, once or twice a week, or many times a day, depending on the woman. Women who go through natural menopause tend to have fewer hot flashes than those whose menopause is surgically induced because the decline of estrogen production is more gradual during natural menopause. Some lucky women never have hot flashes at all—probably because they happen to be good at making estrogen from other sources, such as fat tissue or male hormones (androgens).

Cardiovascular Disease

As estrogen levels decrease, total blood cholesterol levels rise, the good HDL cholesterol decreases, and the bad LDL cholesterol increases. The blood vessels narrow, decreasing the blood flow to heart and brain, and the insides of the arteries become more likely to develop plaque. The lack of progesterone, which helps normalize blood clotting and protect against strokes, may also increase the risk of heart attacks and strokes.

Osteoporosis

After about age 35, women slowly begin to lose the strength and density of their bones. During the years following menopause, the drop-off of estrogen dramatically accelerates the process of bone loss, while the lack of progesterone slows the process of bone rebuilding. The ability to absorb and retain calcium diminishes, making bones more brittle and likely to break. Your chances of fracturing a bone increase greatly and keep rising the older you get. "Crush fractures" of the spine due to calcium loss in the vertebrae, wrist fractures, and hip fractures are the most common osteoporosis-related injuries.

Emotional Changes

A lack of estrogen causes a decrease in levels of endorphins, the body's own natural painkiller and mood elevator. Fewer endorphins translates to more pain, irritability, anxiety, and depression. Progesterone acts as a natural antidepressant, relieves anxiety, and helps normalize blood sugar, so a lack of this hormone may bring on the opposite results.

Mental Changes

Estrogen stimulates the growth of the brain cells, particularly in the cerebral cortex and hypothalamus. It also promotes the growth of nerve cell extensions and helps the nerve cells and the brain link up. An estrogen deficiency can cause memory problems and foggy thinking (which can also result from lack of sleep, another side effect of menopause).

Vaginal Dryness/Infections

The decline of estrogen leads to the shrinkage of the reproductive organs—the vagina, cervix, uterus, and ovaries. The vagina loses muscle tone and its lining gets thinner, drier, and less resilient, making it more likely to tear during intercourse and become infected. Vaginal and cervical mucus production decrease, and changes in the acid-base balance increase the likelihood of bacterial infections.

Incontinence/Urinary Tract Infections

The bladder depends on estrogen to help maintain its muscle tone and elasticity. When estrogen production declines, the bladder becomes weak and flabby, making it less able to hold urine. You may feel an urge to urinate even when there's only a little urine present. At the same time, the muscles that support the pelvic organs begin to lose tone and may allow the urethra to sag. This makes you more prone to urine leakage when you cough, sneeze, or engage in high-impact activities (a condition called *stress incontinence*).

Decline in Sex Drive

Some women may experience a loss of libido due to vaginal dryness, which causes pain during intercourse. On the other hand, many women actually experience an increase in sex drive due to an increase in the ratio of testosterone to both estrogen and progesterone. Testosterone (the male hormone responsible for libido) is produced primarily in the ovaries, so if the ovaries have been removed, this increase in sex drive probably won't occur.

Insomnia

Women who are deficient in estrogen generally take longer to fall asleep, wake up more easily and more often during the night, and spend less time in beneficial REM sleep than those who are not estrogen deficient. Hot flashes, or night sweats, are also major causes of interrupted sleep.

Menopause Is Not a Disease

It's important to remember that even though menopause can produce a laundry list of symptoms, almost nobody suffers from all of them. Also, some of these symptoms are temporary. Hot flashes, night sweats, insomnia, and emotional changes will probably disappear on their own if you give them time.

Some symptoms—such as high total and LDL cholesterol, high blood pressure, atherosclerosis, or osteoporosis—are more troubling, since they can pose serious threats to your health. For the past three decades the medical community's pat answer has been HRT. But today we know that this isn't the solution. So what is? What's actually been proven to help fight the symptoms of menopause, whether they're life threatening or merely annoyances? To find out, I searched the medical literature thoroughly, and what you'll find in the following chapters are the solutions that have been clinically tested and scientifically proven to work.

Chapter Three

Cardiovascular Disease and Hormones

A heart attack or stroke is probably the *last* thing you're worried about. Those things only happen to old people or super-stressed, overweight male business executives in their fifties or sixties—and that's certainly not you. You still have years to go before you need to worry about this kind of thing, right? Wrong. Once you go through menopause, your risk of suffering a heart attack or stroke jumps way up. And after the age of 65, your risk of developing cardiovascular disease (CVD) will equal or exceed that of men. About 480,000 women die annually from CVD, more fatalities than are due to the next fourteen causes of death combined.[1] So you really need to start thinking about how to protect yourself *now*.

CVD is the leading cause of death in American women; almost *half* of us will eventually succumb to it.[2] One in nine women between the ages of 45 and 64 already has some form of heart or blood vessel disease, and women are nearly twice as likely as men to develop the disease at some point in their lives.[3]

Among those women who have heart attacks, a full 42 percent die within the following year.[4] So cardiovascular disease is nothing to fool with. Yet most women appear to be unworried about it, with less than 20 percent even aware that heart disease is a major cause of female death.[5] When I've asked women what worries them most about menopause, they inevitably say "hot flashes" or "moodiness." Almost nobody says "heart disease" or "strokes."

What Is CVD?

Cardiovascular disease can be simply defined as "the dysfunction of the heart and blood vessels," but it's a lot more complex than that. A multifaceted disease, CVD can take the form of high cholesterol, high blood pressure, coronary artery disease, atherosclerosis, congestive heart failure, a heart attack, or a stroke. It generally starts with damage done to the lining of an artery, the blood vessel that carries nutrients and oxygen to the tissues (as opposed to a vein, which carries waste products away from the tissues). The damaged site provides a perfect place for the buildup of *plaque*, a thick, waxy substance made up of fat, cholesterol, smooth muscle cells, and other cellular debris.

Atherosclerosis

This accumulation of plaque causes a chronic disease called *atherosclerosis*, in which the artery walls become thick, hard, and stiff. It's important for arteries to be able to expand and contract on command so they can divert blood to the areas that need it. But atherosclerotic arteries lose their elasticity and stay permanently narrowed, like little concrete tubes. The buildup of plaque can eventually choke off the blood supply to tissues and organs, setting the stage for a heart attack or stroke. The four things that are most likely to bring on atherosclerosis are smoking, high cholesterol (total or LDL), high blood pressure, and lack of physical activity, although high levels of iron, diabetes, and obesity can also play a part.

Thick, Sticky Blood

While atherosclerosis is a case of artery walls that are too thick and sticky, blood that's too thick or sticky can be just as great a problem. While it's absolutely necessary for your blood to clot when you've been injured, if your blood is so full of clotting substances that it doesn't slide through your blood vessels easily or it clots too quickly, blockages are more likely to form. Almost all heart attacks are the result of atherosclerosis in the coronary arteries coupled with one or more clots. Strokes, on the other hand, can be the result of either a clot or a hemmorhage in an artery that serves the brain.

It All Begins with a Scratch

In the past, experts believed that arterial plaque simply built up to the point where it choked off the blood supply, or a piece of plaque or a blood clot floated through the bloodstream until it got caught in a smaller blood vessel and formed a blockage. While these scenarios are possible, many experts now believe that most CVD begins with a little injury to the lining of an artery.

Many things can cause this little scratch, including a certain kind of cholesterol (LDL), high blood pressure, smoking, free radicals, infections, or diabetes.

Whatever the cause, once the arterial lining is scratched, the body goes into overdrive, triggering the inflammation process and sending immune system cells to attempt to patch things up. But the repair process is anything but perfect, and some of the immune system cells end up burrowing into the artery wall itself. There they produce adhesion molecules, sticky substances that encourage other cells to join them. Cholesterol, fat cells, smooth muscle cells, connective tissue cells, and substances that make the blood clot are immediately attracted to the area like ants to a glob of honey. Soon the inside of the wall is "pregnant" with a big, fatty conglomeration of cells that have the ability to trigger an instantaneous blood clot.

A Little Ticking "Time Bomb"

This combination of cells takes up residence in the wall of the artery, where it forms a little ticking "time bomb." The body senses the presence of a dangerous enemy and forms a tough, fibrous cap to seal it off. But the artery lining remains forever changed once a "time bomb" has been implanted, becoming much more likely to encourage plaque formation. In other words, once a "time bomb" forms in an artery, you'll be a lot more likely to clog up your arteries and form more "time bombs." Then it's just a matter of time before one of them explodes.

The explosion countdown begins when the fibrous cap wears away, eroded by the constant flow of blood. Then the contents of the "time bomb" spill into the bloodstream and form a huge clot, thanks to their high-powered clotting substances. The clot instantly fills the artery and blocks it completely, triggering a heart attack (if the artery serves the heart) or a stroke (if the artery serves the brain).

These "time bombs" are often completely buried in an artery wall and don't protrude into the bloodstream or block the artery at all until they rupture. That's why some people with completely clear arteries and no obvious symptoms of CVD end up having heart attacks or strokes, while others with arteries that are 80 percent blocked manage to live for years with no trouble.

There are some other ways of triggering a heart attack or a stroke. A heart attack can be caused by a sudden, prolonged spasm in an artery serving the heart, while a stroke can result from the rupture of a blood vessel that feeds the brain. But the majority of heart attacks and strokes are caused by blockages, and it's likely that many of them are triggered by the spillage of the contents of a "time bomb" into the bloodstream.

Risk Factors for Cardiovascular Disease

Cardiovascular disease can be brought on or made worse by many things, some of which you can change, and some of which you can't.

Things You Can Change

- *High blood pressure (hypertension)*—If you've got high blood pressure, the insides of your blood vessels are taking a real beating, even though you probably won't have any symptoms that indicate this. This pressure increases the likelihood of arterial injuries (scratches), plaque formation, permanently narrowed arteries, and

Symptoms of Cardiovascular Disease

Cardiovascular disease is a gradual process that can progress for decades before any obvious symptoms arise, but it can produce two potentially devastating outcomes: a heart attack or a stroke.

Heart Attack

There are no symptoms in the early stages of heart disease. People can still function well with coronary arteries that are almost completely blocked. When symptoms finally do strike, they may include:

- angina—chest pain usually related to exertion that can radiate to the shoulders and arms, neck and jaw, the upper abdomen, shoulders, or back
- a "crushing" or "squeezing" feeling in the chest
- shortness of breath, light-headedness
- sweating, nausea
- fatigue, fainting

Stroke

A major cause of disability or death, stroke symptoms will depend upon which area of the brain is affected. Symptoms may gradually grow worse over a period of hours or days and can include:

- sudden weakness or numbness affecting one side of the body, particularly the face, arm, or leg
- difficulty speaking or understanding speech, or loss of speech
- partial or complete loss of vision, double vision

- dizziness, loss of balance, falling
- transient ischemic attacks (TIAs)—"small" strokes that occur when an artery that serves the brain is temporarily clogged; symptoms are similar to those of a major stroke, but they're temporary and on a much smaller scale

blood clots. High blood pressure is the number one risk factor for stroke.

- *Elevated total cholesterol*—Too much cholesterol in the blood contributes to the clogging of the arteries via the deposition of fatty substances within artery walls ("time bombs").
- *Elevated LDL (bad) cholesterol*—Low-density lipoproteins are called the "bad" cholesterol because they tend to leave fatty deposits on artery walls, leading to plaque formation and heart disease.
- *Low HDL (good) cholesterol*—High-density lipoproteins are called the "good" cholesterol because they carry cholesterol out of the arteries to the liver, where it's processed for excretion. So the more HDL, the better.
- *Smoking*—Cigarette smoking damages artery linings, raises LDL cholesterol, lowers HDL cholesterol, narrows the arteries and reduces their ability to deliver oxygen to the tissues, encourages early menopause due to lowered estrogen levels, and increases the likelihood of clot formation, coronary spasms, and erratic heart rhythms.
- *Obesity*—Excess weight puts a strain on the heart and increases the risk of heart disease, especially if fat accumulates in the abdominal

area. Abdominal obesity is also linked to high levels of blood fats (cholesterol, triglycerides), hypertension, and Type II diabetes.

- *Stress*—Stress increases blood pressure, heart rate, the level of fats in the blood, blood vessel constriction, and the tendency of the blood to clot, all of which can increase the risk of heart attacks or strokes.
- *Lack of exercise*—People who lead sedentary lives tend to be overweight, have higher total cholesterol and LDL, lower HDL, higher blood pressure, and a higher risk of becoming diabetic. Regular exercise burns fat, raises HDL, lowers LDL and other blood fats, strengthens the cardiovascular system, and improves overall health. Those who exercise regularly are much less likely to have heart attacks or strokes.

Things You Can't Change

- *Family history of heart disease or stroke*—Your risk of heart attack or stroke increases if either of your parents had heart or blood vessel disease, particularly if developed before the age of 55.
- *Ethnicity*—Black women are more at risk of CVD than white women up until age 75. Strokes are also more common among African Americans.
- *Gender*—Men are more than twice as likely as women to have a stroke. As for heart disease, the death rate is higher for men than for women, particularly in the 35 to 55 age range. But after age 55, the death rate for men falls, and rises for women.
- *Age*—The risk of cardiovascular disease rises

with age. One in nine women between the ages of 45 and 64 has CVD, but at age 65 the risk rises to one in three. Age is also associated with an increased risk of hypertension, high cholesterol, being overweight, and diabetes.

- *Being postmenopausal*—The decline in estrogen production accompanying menopause results in higher total cholesterol, higher LDL, lower HDL, narrowing of the arteries due to plaque deposition, and arterial stiffening due to a decreased ability to dilate.

- *Existing heart disease*—Once you've had a heart attack, you're twice as likely to have another one. And existing heart disease will make you more than twice as likely to have a stroke than a woman without heart disease.

- *Diabetes mellitus*—Diabetes promotes the deposition of plaque on artery walls, damages artery linings, drives up blood fats, and doubles your risk of heart attack. If you're diabetic, it's essential to keep your blood sugar under control to ward off CVD.

The Estrogen–Cardiovascular Disease Connection

In July 2001, an entire year before the WHI study was called to a screeching halt, the American Heart Association reversed their long-held position about HRT. Suddenly they started recommending that women *not* be given hormone replacement therapy if the only reason for doing so was to prevent heart disease. Why the unexpected turnaround? Because evidence was piling up that HRT was not the magic pill that everyone thought it was. The results of the most recent studies of HRT's effect on the heart and blood vessels had been lukewarm at best, if not downright negative. So the American Heart Association finally felt compelled to withdraw its support of HRT—a complete turnaround from the position they'd held for years.

But it wasn't just the American Heart Association that had been on the HRT bandwagon. The American Medical Association, the American College of Cardiology, the American College of Obstetricians and Gynecologists, and many other big guns had long recommended that HRT at least be considered for *all* postmenopausal women, since its heart protective effects seemed so obvious. And, indeed, there were plenty of reasons for them to think this way. CVD rarely appears in women until after menopause, but as soon as menopause sets in, a woman's risk will rise until it equals that of a man. Why? Experts believe it's due to the loss of the cardioprotective effect of estrogen.

And there are other indications of a link between hormones and cardiovascular disease:

- Although age plays a part in heart disease, it appears to be less important than menopausal status. When looking at women of the *same age*, those who are postmenopausal will tend to have significantly higher rates of heart disease than those who are premenopausal.
- Women who go through menopause early (whether it's natural or induced surgically) are more likely to develop premature heart disease.
- Autopsies of women who had their ovaries removed and didn't take estrogen replacement show an increase in the progression of heart dis-

ease when compared with women who still had their ovaries.

- Total cholesterol and LDL cholesterol increase sharply at menopause when estrogen levels drop, and rise until at least age 60, when they stabilize at this higher level.
- HDL cholesterol decreases as estrogen levels drop.
- High blood pressure, a major risk factor for cardiovascular disease, is much more prevalent in postmenopausal women, striking more than half of women over age 55.

Estrogen Replacement: The Pros

But when estrogen levels were restored through HRT, the heart protective effects seemed to come back, as well. Various studies have found that estrogen:

- lowers total cholesterol
- lowers LDL
- raises HDL
- protects blood vessel linings from scratches
- helps the blood vessels relax and widen, which decreases blood pressure
- decreases fibrinogen, a protein essential to the blood clotting process, so it lessens the risk of clot formation
- improves insulin sensitivity, so insulin levels decline (too much insulin damages the insides of the arteries and may be the first step in the progression toward a heart attack)

Estrogen Replacement: The Cons

But the news wasn't all good. There were negative findings, too:

- In 1995, the Postmenopausal Estrogen/Progestin Interventions (PEPI) trial reported that estrogen increased both inflammation and the levels of triglycerides (fats) in the blood—bad news for the heart.[6]
- In older postmenopausal women who'd had recent heart attacks, HRT increased the risk of blood clots.[7]
- Although estrogen replacement was associated with a lower risk of heart attack in women who entered menopause before age 55, this was not seen in women who went through menopause after age 55.[8]
- The Heart and Estrogen/Progestin Replacement Study (HERS) found that estrogen did *nothing* to reduce a woman's risk of heart attack or coronary death. In fact, women with heart disease who took HRT were even a bit *more* likely to have a heart attack, at least during the first couple years of therapy.[9]
- The Estrogen Replacement and Atherosclerosis trial (ERA) showed that HRT did nothing to control the buildup of plaque inside the heart's arteries. HRT also increased the incidence of blood clots and gallbladder disease, and slightly increased the levels of triglycerides (blood fats).[10]

Is It Good or Is It Bad?

So now what? We had a boatload of studies saying that HRT did all kinds of wonderful things for the heart and the blood vessels. Then along came a bunch more saying it was either bad for the heart or not nearly as protective as we'd been led to believe. What were we supposed to think?

In order to understand the importance of what happened next, you need to realize that there hadn't been enough time to figure out whether or not women who went on HRT when they were 50 would actually have fewer heart attacks or strokes five or more years down the road. Researchers had only looked at the indicators of heart disease, then guessed how they might translate into actual cardiovascular events. We needed a long-term, randomized, placebo-controlled trial of HRT on a very large group of women to see how it really affected them. Thus, the mega-importance of the Women's Health Initiative (WHI) study, which was begun in 1997. Finally, we were going to get some definitive answers.

The WHI study was comprised of a series of large, population-based trials testing the risks and benefits of different strategies for protecting the health of more than 16,000 women who had already gone through menopause. In July 2002, three years before the scheduled end of the study, the researchers already knew enough: HRT was dangerous, causing a slight but significant increase in the risk of heart attacks, blood clots, strokes, and breast cancer.

So how come 2 + 2 didn't add up to 4? Why such positive results on the indicators of CVD and negative results in the long term? No one is really sure. It should be noted that the hormone replacement used in the trial was PREMPRO—a combination of synthetic estrogen and synthetic progesterone. Other forms of hormones (natural ones, those with different combinations, or those with different delivery systems) might possibly bring about different results.

But for the time being, HRT doesn't appear to be a viable answer to the CVD problem.

What We Really Need

Whether hormone replacement works or doesn't work, all of us postmenopausal women need the same thing: something to keep our cholesterol (particularly the LDL) low, our blood pressure within normal range, and our arteries flexible. If we can do these things, we can dramatically lower our risk of having a heart attack or stroke. And luckily there are plenty of natural methods—all backed by solid scientific studies proving their effectiveness—that can help us do just that.

Chapter Four

Cholesterol: The Good, the Bad, and the Ugly

Contrary to what you've probably heard for years, cholesterol is actually a *good* thing. A waxy, fatty substance used to make cell membranes and to insulate nerves, cholesterol plays an important part in the manufacture of estrogen, testosterone, the active vitamin D hormone, and the fat-digesting bile acids. But experts have known for decades that too much cholesterol floating through your bloodstream is linked to the clogging of the arteries, heart disease, heart attacks, and strokes.

Your body makes about three-quarters of its cholesterol supply, and the rest comes from what you eat. So you *do* have some control over how high your cholesterol rises. Eating a diet high in saturated fat and cholesterol can send your cholesterol levels soaring, while a diet low in these kinds of foods can bring blood cholesterol back down to a healthier range.

The Problem

Too much total cholesterol and LDL contribute to atherosclerosis, a buildup of plaque in the arteries that makes them more likely to become blocked. Depending upon where a blockage occurs, it may cause a heart attack or a stroke. Total cholesterol levels over 200 mg/dL and LDL levels over 130 mg/dL increase your risk of cardiovascular disease, while HDL levels over 40 mg/dL are protective. When estrogen levels drop at menopause, total cholesterol and LDL tend to rise, while HDL tends to drop.

Kinds of Cholesterol

Cholesterol takes several forms inside your body, and each form has different properties. It makes sense, then, that each would be measured separately. For our purposes, however, we'll just look at the three most common cholesterol measurements: *total cholesterol*, *LDL*, and *HDL*.

Total Cholesterol

When people ask you what your cholesterol level is, they mean your total cholesterol level, which is a blanket measurement of all the cholesterol in your bloodstream. As total cholesterol increases, so does your risk of atherosclerosis, heart disease, heart attack, and stroke. In fact, a large-scale study following 325,000 healthy men for 10 years found that those who had total cholesterol levels of over 300 mg/dL had almost five times the risk of dying of heart disease than those with levels below 180 mg/dL.[1]

According to the American Heart Association, the ideal level of total cholesterol falls somewhere between 130 mg/dL and 190 mg/dL, and levels over 200 mg/dL show increased risk. A total cholesterol level of 300 mg/dL doubles your chances of having a heart attack.

Low-Density Lipoproteins (LDL)

Low-density lipoproteins (LDL) are the primary carriers of cholesterol to the organs and tissues that need it. Since cholesterol can't just float around the body by itself, it attaches itself to a protein molecule, which gives it a ride through the bloodstream. But LDL tends to leave fatty deposits on the walls of the arteries along the way, narrowing their passageways and reducing the flow of blood. That's why it's often called the "bad" cholesterol. If you have high levels of LDL, that means you have lots of cholesterol floating through your bloodstream, just looking for trouble.

LDL becomes particularly dangerous when it's been *oxidized*, a chemical process that occurs within the body and makes LDL more likely to stick to artery walls. Oxidized LDL is irritating to the artery wall and can actually wound it, causing the scratch that starts the process of atherosclerosis. LDL levels typically increase after menopause, which may be the reason that the risk of CVD is higher in postmenopausal women. A diet high in saturated fat increases LDL, but genetics play a role too, with some people clearing the LDL and fats from their bloodstreams more quickly than others. Ideally, your LDL levels should be below 130 mg/dL.

High-Density Lipoproteins (HDL)

High-density lipoproteins (HDL) are the body's cholesterol scavengers, carrying cholesterol away from artery walls and to the liver for excretion. HDL acts as a sort of cholesterol clean-up molecule, so the higher your HDL, the lower your risk of heart disease. Conversely, a low level of HDL is a dangerous sign. Even if your total cholesterol and LDL aren't high, a low HDL level will increase your risk of atherosclerosis, heart attacks, and strokes because cholesterol is allowed to build up. Like LDL, your HDL level may be determined in part by genetics, but it will drop after menopause. A high-fat diet, obesity, smoking, or a sedentary lifestyle will also lower your HDL significantly, while regular exercise can do much to increase it. Ideally, your HDL should be above 40 mg/dL. Levels lower than 35 mg/dL can double your heart attack risk.

Total Cholesterol Divided by HDL—A More Accurate Assessment of CVD Risk

Just knowing your total cholesterol, LDL, and HDL numbers won't be enough to paint an accurate picture of your cardiovascular disease risk. What's most important is the ratio of total cholesterol to HDL. To find this ratio, divide your total cholesterol by your HDL. (For example, if your total cholesterol is 166 mg/dL and your HDL is 40 mg/dL, divide 166 by 40. The answer is 4.15.)

If your answer is less than 4.5, you're doing well. If it's over 5.0, you're at risk for a heart attack or stroke.

Estrogen and Cholesterol

Estrogen helps protect premenopausal women from heart disease by keeping total cholesterol and LDL on the low side, while giving HDL a boost. But when estrogen levels drop at menopause, its protective effect is lost, allowing total cholesterol and LDL to rise while the beneficial HDL dwindles. Because of these hormone-driven changes in cholesterol, the risk of cardiovascular disease in postmenopausal women increases, eventually equaling that of men. Luckily, just lowering your total cholesterol levels can significantly reduce your risk of cardiovascular disease. In populations where the average total cholesterol level is less than 160 mg/dL, CVD doesn't even exist.[2]

In General, You Want To:

- keep your total cholesterol below 200 mg/dL
- keep your LDL below 130 mg/dL
- keep your HDL over 40 mg/dL
- prevent the oxidation of your LDL
- keep your blood "thin" to help prevent the formation of deadly clots

What You Can Do About It

Diet

Adopt a Mediterranean-Style Diet
Originating in the countries that border the Mediterranean Sea, such as Italy and Greece, the Mediterranean-style diet features plenty of fresh fruits and vegetables (both green and root), nuts and cereals, olives, olive oil, fish, and cheese, and moderate amounts of wine (although it's optional). There's a lot less cardiovascular disease in countries favoring the Mediterranean diet compared to those that follow the standard Western diet, even though the total fat intake in the Mediterranean diet is substantial (35 percent of total calories). But much of the fat in the diet comes from olive oil, a monounsaturated fat,

which is known to lower total cholesterol and LDL, while reducing the oxidation of LDL. Red wine may also play a part. (See section on red wine, page 55.)

A great deal of research suggests that adopting a low saturated fat, high fiber, high complex carbohydrate diet like this can lower the cholesterol and blood fats by some 20 percent.[3] And since the risk of heart disease drops 2 percent with every 1 percent drop in total cholesterol, this diet alone may be able to reduce your risk of heart disease by as much as 40 percent.[4]

Recommendation: Eat more like an Italian! Use olive oil as your main source of fat and have plenty of pasta, potatoes, and whole grains. Eat a salad with an olive oil–based dressing with every meal. Emphasize fruits and vegetables, while scaling back on meat. Substitute red wine for other alcoholic beverages, if you drink them.

Reduce Saturated Fat/Cholesterol Intake

A diet high in saturated fat raises blood cholesterol levels more than anything else. Finns, who eat more saturated fat than any other national group, also have the highest cholesterol levels and the highest rates of heart disease.[5] But the opposite relationship is also true: lowering your saturated fat intake can result in a marked decrease in your blood cholesterol levels.

Saturated fats are generally found in animal products and tend to be solid at room temperature (think butter and lard). Most experts recommend that our saturated fat intake provide no more than about 10 percent of our daily calories. Unfortunately, most Americans are getting much more of this artery-clogging fat in their diets, which is reflected in our current worldwide status as the country with the highest levels of heart disease—after Finland.

The effect of cholesterol intake from foods can be mixed. Although most people can consume cholesterol without it affecting their blood cholesterol levels, some people are cholesterol sensitive and have a problem if they eat cholesterol-containing foods. For this reason, the American Heart Association and other experts recommend a low cholesterol intake. Also, foods high in cholesterol are often high in saturated fat, which *will* raise blood cholesterol. So unless you know that you're not cholesterol sensitive, it may be better to stay away from high-cholesterol foods.

Recommendation: Cut way back on your saturated fat intake, substituting monounsaturated fats (such as olive oil or canola oil) whenever possible. The main sources of saturated fat in the American diet include red meat, whole milk, cheese, processed meats, poultry skin, ice cream, and baked goods. Limit high-cholesterol foods such as eggs, red meats, organ meats, shellfish, and most animal products, unless you're sure you're not cholesterol sensitive.

Limit Trans-Fatty Acids

Trans-fatty acids (TFAs) are created when unsaturated fats are altered to make them act like saturated ones. An example of this is margarine. Manufacturers take liquid vegetable oil and add hydrogen, and— voilà!—the liquid becomes a solid you can spread on your bread. Hydrogenated fats act like saturated fats in your body, but they're even worse. That's because between 8 and 70 percent of them take on a different configuration, creating a kind of "fake fat" seldom seen in nature—the trans-fatty acid. TFAs raise LDL levels, increase inflammation, and elevate total cholesterol. When scientists at Harvard Medical School looked at the diets of 85,095 healthy women, they found that the more TFAs the women had in their diet, the higher their risk of developing cardiovascular disease.[6]

Recommendation: Lower your intake of TFAs. You can do this by avoiding fast food, fried food, and foods that contain hydrogenated or partially hydrogenated vegetable oil. Diet margarine or margarines that clearly state "no trans-fatty acids" on the label are your best bets for spreads.

Foods and Phytochemicals

Although diet is key to controlling cholesterol levels, certain individual foods or components of food called *phytochemicals* (literally, "plant chemicals") can also be of help. Remember, though, that none of these are stand-alone solutions to the problem of heart disease. Your overall diet and lifestyle are far more important to reducing your risk of CVD than any single food or supplement.

Bioflavonoids

The bioflavonoids are a group of more than 200 substances found in the outer layers, skin, and peel of vegetables and fruits, in leafy green vegetables, and in coffee, tea, and wine that act as powerful antioxidants. Some common bioflavonoids are hesperidin, rutin, quercetin, and catechin. Besides their antioxidant properties, they can help "thin" the blood[7] (preventing the formation of potentially deadly blood clots) and fight the oxidation of LDL.

Recommendation: Eat five or more servings of vegetables and fruits daily.

Coenzyme Q10

Coenzyme Q10 (also known as CoQ10 or ubiquinone) is found everywhere in foods and in the body, where it plays an important role in energy production. CoQ10 is a strong antioxidant that can help reduce total cholesterol and LDL cholesterol, fight LDL oxidation, decrease the heart rate, improve oxygen delivery, and possibly even improve heart function.[8] CoQ10 deficiencies have been seen in some cases of heart disease.[9]

- Japanese researchers found that heart patients had lower ratios of CoQ10 to total cholesterol and LDL than people without heart disease. This suggests that a lack of CoQ10 may encourage high total cholesterol and LDL—or that higher levels of CoQ10 protect against atherosclerosis and heart disease by decreasing total cholesterol and LDL.[10]
- CoQ10 has been used to relieve the symptoms of angina, which is caused by the dangerous narrowing of coronary arteries and the subsequent strain it places on the heart. When men and women with angina were given either CoQ10 or a placebo for 4 weeks, those who took CoQ10 had 53 percent fewer angina episodes and were able to exercise longer on a treadmill.[11]
- CoQ10 may also help to reduce the risk of heart disease by keeping the blood "thin."[12]

Caution: Taking CoQ10 supplements may cause gastritis, nausea, diarrhea, or lack of appetite and could reduce the effectiveness of blood thinners.

Recommendation: Typical doses are 50–100 mg of CoQ10 twice a day.

Garlic (Allium sativum)

In ancient times, the famous physician Dioscorides recorded that this strong-smelling vegetable could help keep the arteries open and the blood flowing freely.[13] Today, studies have found that garlic can help lower cholesterol and protect against heart disease by thinning the blood, lowering both total and LDL cholesterol, and raising HDL cholesterol.

- Researchers in India studied 432 heart disease patients, half of whom received a glass of milk containing the juice of 6–10 grams of garlic each morning. In the garlic group, the overall death rate was reduced by 50 percent during the second year and the heart attack rate had decreased 60 percent by the third year. In addition, blood cholesterol, blood pressure, and joint pain decreased, while energy increased.[14]
- A combined review of several studies showed that eating one half to one clove of garlic daily reduced total cholesterol by 8 percent and triglycerides by 13 percent, a result that lasted for six months or longer.[15]
- One study found that 600 mg of garlic powder a day can push total cholesterol down by some 10 percent, which translates to a 20 percent decrease in the risk of heart disease.[16]

Recommendation: Add garlic to your food whenever possible, eating up to three cloves per day. Use liberally in stir-fries, soups, salads, or casseroles. Or try roasting it wrapped in foil at 350 degrees for 45 minutes, then squeeze the juice on bread.

Gugulipid (Commiphora mukul)

A tree resin that's been used as an Indian folk remedy for 2,000 years, gugulipid (also known as guggul) blocks the recycling of bile acids, which are made from cholesterol. Then cholesterol in the blood must be used to manufacture new bile, effectively lowering circulating cholesterol levels. Gugulipid may also inhibit the liver's production of cholesterol, stimulate the thyroid gland, promote weight loss, and reduce blood fats.[17]

- The effects of 50 mg of gugulipid taken twice a day for 24 weeks was tested in 61 people with elevated cholesterol. Half were given gugulipid, the others a placebo, and everyone ate a diet rich in fruits and vegetables. Those taking the gugulipid decreased their total cholesterol by an average 11.7 percent, their LDL by 12.5 percent, and their triglycerides by 12 percent.[18]
- Another study involved more than 200 people taking 500 mg of guggul gum three times a day for 12 weeks. Taking the guggul gum caused total cholesterol to fall 22 percent and the blood fats by 25 percent.[19]
- The *Journal of Associated Physicians—India* published a study in which 125 people took gugulipid. In 3 to 4 weeks, they saw their total cholesterol levels and blood fats fall by an average of 11 percent and 16 percent, respectively, and their HDLs rise an average of 60 percent.[20]

Caution: Mild nausea, hiccups, headache, or skin rash can result from taking gugulipid. It may also interfere with the action of certain heart or blood pressure medicines. Consult your physician before taking.

Recommendation: A daily dose of 50–500 mg of gugulipid for at least 24 weeks has been used to lower cholesterol.

Oat Bran

Oat bran, a fiber found in oats that dissolves in water, helps reduce total cholesterol and LDL cholesterol when it's consumed as part of a low-saturated-fat and low-cholesterol diet.[21] It works primarily by sopping up excess cholesterol and fatty acids in the intestines and speeding them out of the body. Like gugulipid, oat bran inhibits the recycling of bile acids. But it also absorbs the bile acids and sends them through the intestines for excretion through the feces. As such, oat bran forces the body to use blood cholesterol to manufacture new bile acids.

- Sixty-six men from northern Mexico with normal or elevated cholesterol levels were enrolled in an 8-week study testing the ability of different kinds of dietary fiber to reduce LDL cholesterol. Those who began the study with elevated cholesterol and blood fats and ate the oat bran were able to lower their LDL cholesterol by 26 percent and blood fats by 28 percent.[22]
- Finnish researchers studied the effects of supplementing the diet with oat bran in men with elevated cholesterol and blood fats. The 59 men were given 70 grams of oat bran per day for 6 weeks and their total cholesterol levels fell an average of 9.5 percent.[23]
- Scientists at the University of California found that adding 84 grams of an oat bran product to the diet every day for 6 weeks reduced total cholesterol an average of 13 percent.[24]

Caution: If you have an allergy to gluten, oat bran can trigger an allergic reaction. Those with bowel problems, or problems chewing or swallowing food, may develop intestinal obstructions. Oat bran can cause intestinal gas, especially if you're not used to eating it. Start with small amounts and increase gradually.

Recommendation: A typical daily dose for reducing cholesterol is 28 grams of oat bran (or about 1 oz). You can sprinkle it on cereal, add it to baked goods, or eat it as a hot cereal by itself. One study found that oat bran lowers cholesterol most effectively in those over the age of 50.[25]

Omega-3 Fatty Acids/Fish

Omega-3 fatty acids are special building blocks of fat found in fish and certain other foods. Scientists have found that the more omega-3s there are in body tissues, the lower the risk of developing CVD.[26] That's because omega-3s can inhibit clot formation, reduce total cholesterol, decrease atherosclerosis, lower the blood fats (triglycerides), and increase HDL cholesterol levels.

- A 16-year study of nearly 85,000 women found that eating fish two to four times a week cut their risk of developing heart disease by 30 percent. And if they ate fish five times a week, their risk dropped by 34 percent.[27]
- Another large-scale study found that eating fish once or twice a week can lower the risk of dying of heart disease by one-half.[28]
- A 17-year study of men who did not have heart disease found that those who had the most omega-3 fatty acids in their blood were 80 percent less likely to die suddenly from heart disease than those who had the least.[29]

The best sources of omega-3 are cold water fish and fish oils. Cold water fish that are good sources of omega-3 include:

- anchovies
- Atlantic sturgeon
- herring
- mackerel
- salmon
- sardines
- trout
- tuna

You can also get omega-3 fatty acids by eating flax products, which contain substances that can be converted to omega-3 fatty acids in the body. However, the conversion process is somewhat inefficient, particularly in the elderly.

Caution: Eating several servings of fish per week probably can't hurt you. But if you take omega-3s in their concentrated form as fish oil, you may experience certain problems:

- Fish oil may cause heartburn, nosebleeds, vitamin E depletion, belching, and halitosis. Large doses may trigger loose stools and nausea.
- Using fish oil with medications or herbs that have anticoagulant or antiplatelet actions could increase the risk of bleeding.
- Fish oil may also interfere with certain antidiabetic and antihypertensive drugs.
- Fish oil should be used with caution if you have diabetes, hypertension, or cirrhosis, or if you are aspirin sensitive.
- Consult your health care provider before taking fish oil.

Recommendation: For heart health, many experts recommend taking 3–4 grams of omega-3 fatty acids per day. You can get this amount by consuming:

- 1.5 oz of cold water fish daily; *or*
- three to five 3-oz servings of cold water fish weekly; *or*
- 1–2 tsp of fish oil daily; *or*
- 3–4 1,000 mg capsules of fish oil daily

Or, if you prefer flaxseed, take:

- 1 tsp of ground flaxseed daily; *or*
- Three to five servings of whole grain products made with flax weekly; *or*
- 1-2 T of flaxseed oil; *or*
- 1–2 omega-3 enriched eggs, which come from hens that are fed ground flaxseed, per week

Policosanol

Policosanol is derived from the sugarcane. Its main ingredient is *octacosanol*, an alcohol found in the waxy coating of fruit and leaves. Studies have shown that policosanol can lower cholesterol by slowing its production in the liver. Policosanol also increases the rate at which LDL cholesterol is broken down, protects against the arterial scratches that can trigger atherosclerosis, and raises HDL better than most of the statins (the current "wonder drugs" for controlling cholesterol levels).

- In a study of 244 postmenopausal women with elevated total cholesterol and LDL cholesterol, daily doses of 5 mg policosanol for 12 weeks lowered total cholesterol by 13 percent and LDL by 18 percent, and increased HDL by 17 percent. When the dose was increased to 10 mg per day, the overall levels of total cholesterol dropped by 17 percent and LDL by 25 percent, while HDL increased by 29 percent.[30]

- Chilean researchers tested policosanol's prowess against two standard cholesterol-lowering medicines, lovastatin and simvastatin, in an 8-week study of 106 patients whose LDL levels were over 160 mg/dL. Policosanol lowered the LDL by 24 percent, compared to lovastatin's 22 percent and simvastatin's 15 percent. It also pushed the HDL cholesterol up, which wasn't seen with either of the drugs.[31]
- Cuban researchers found that taking 10 mg of policosanol per day for 30 days lowered platelet aggregation (the tendency of the blood to clot).[32] Blood tests given to 37 healthy volunteers who took increasing doses of policosanol revealed that the greater the dose of policosanol, the greater the antiplatelet effects.[33]

Caution: Oral doses of up to 10 mg per day, taken for up to 24 months, are "possibly safe." Oral policosanol may trigger migraines, insomnia, irritability, and other side effects. Policosanol has antiplatelet effects, so in theory it might increase the risk of bleeding in those taking aspirin or other substances that thin the blood.

Recommendation: A typical dose of policosanol is 5 mg twice daily.

Red Wine

For decades, doctors have been baffled by the "French paradox," the fact that the French eat a high-fat diet yet their incidence of heart disease is 50 percent less than that of Americans. The French also smoke more than we do, and are probably just as stressed. So what protects French hearts? The answer may be red wine, or more specifically, the polyphenol that's present in red wine, *resveratrol*. While alcohol in general has gained a reputation over the past 20 years for being cardioprotective, red wine may lead the pack when it comes to preventing atherosclerosis and helping the heart stay healthy due to red wine's polyphenol content.

- A review of large population studies on alcohol consumption and various disease states performed over the past 20 years found that red wine has high levels of phenolic compounds (including resveratrol) that increase HDL, antioxidant activity, and the widening of the arteries, while discouraging formation of clots, clumping of the platelets, and platelets' ability to stick to artery walls.[34]
- In laboratory experiments, researchers added red wine to human LDL and found that the resveratrol in the wine inhibited the oxidation of LDL significantly—by 60 percent in one trial and 98 percent in another.[35]
- Results from a study done by British scientists in 2001 suggest that red wine may fight heart disease because its polyphenols block a protein called endothelin-1 (ET-1) that's involved in the formation of fatty streaks in blood vessels, an early sign of heart disease, and the constriction of blood vessels. The red wine that appeared to suppress ET-1 the most was cabernet sauvignon.[36]

Caution: While regular consumption of about one 6 oz. glass of red wine per day may help protect the cardiovascular system, consumption of more may increase the risk of heart disease, breast cancer, and alcoholism.[37]

Recommendation: If you don't drink, don't start now

to protect your heart. But if you do enjoy a glass of wine and you're not a problem drinker, a little red wine with dinner may be helpful.

Red Yeast Rice (Monascus purpureus)

Also known as *zhithai* or *xuezhikang*, red yeast rice is created by growing red yeast on rice, then fermenting it. It's been used in China for cooking and medicinal purposes since the ninth century. Red yeast rice contains a small amount of an ingredient that's chemically identical to lovastatin, one of the statin family of cholesterol-lowering drugs, which works by inhibiting cholesterol production in the liver. In 1998, the Food and Drug Administration ruled that red yeast rice was a drug because of its chemical makeup. The decision has since been overruled, making red yeast rice difficult to find in the stores. But it is still available via the Internet and may be worthwhile to look into if you have high cholesterol. Tests conducted on both animals and humans have shown promising results:

- Modern Chinese studies on animals show that red yeast rice can reduce total cholesterol by 11 to 32 percent and blood fats (triglycerides) by 12 to 19 percent.[38]
- A 12-week study of 46 men and 37 women with elevated cholesterol, all of whom followed a low-fat, low-cholesterol diet, showed significant reductions in total cholesterol, LDL cholesterol, and blood fats in those who took red yeast rice, compared to those who did not.[39]
- Chinese researchers tested a red yeast rice preparation in 324 people with elevated cholesterol. After 8 weeks, total cholesterol levels had fallen

an average of 23 percent, while HDL cholesterol had risen by 20 percent.[40]

Caution: Side effects may include gastric distress or elevated liver enzymes. Since red yeast rice contains an ingredient identical to lovastatin, it should not be used in conjunction with the statin drugs or any other drugs to lower cholesterol. People who have or are at risk of developing liver dysfunction should avoid red yeast rice.

Recommendation: A standard dose for lowering elevated cholesterol is 600 mg of red yeast rice taken two to four times a day with food. Consult your health care provider before taking red yeast rice.

Soy or Soybeans

A popular food in Japan and other Asian countries, soy contains good amounts of fiber, calcium, iron, potassium, and other nutrients. Here in the United States, we eat soy in the form of soybeans, soy flour, soy milk, soy oil, tofu, miso, tempeh, natto, and other foods. Soy contains *phytoestrogens* (literally, "plant estrogens") that have mild estrogenlike effects on the body. During and after menopause, when declining estrogen levels bring about a decrease in HDL and an increase in LDL, eating soy or soy products may help improve these cholesterol levels. The phytoestrogens in soy come in the form of *isoflavones*, which are antioxidants that help protect the body from free radical damage and oxidation.

- A study reported in the *American Journal of Clinical Nutrition* in August 2002, involving 41 men and postmenopausal women with high cholesterol and blood fats, found that substituting soy foods for animal products reduced blood fats and oxidized LDL, and lowered blood pressure.[41]

- A 1995 meta analysis published in the *New England Journal of Medicine* that looked at the combined results of 38 studies found that consuming 47 grams of soy protein daily leads to a 9.3 percent drop in total cholesterol, a 12.9 percent drop in the dangerous LDL cholesterol, a 10.5 percent fall in triglycerides (blood fats), and a 2.4 percent increase in the helpful HDL cholesterol. The authors concluded that simply adding soy protein to the diet could lower heart disease risk by 20 to 30 percent.[42]

- Another study looked at the link between consumption of dietary phytoestrogens and cardiovascular risk in 403 postmenopausal women. The results showed that dietary phytoestrogens can protect against atherosclerosis and the stiffening of the aorta, and that older women are especially likely to benefit.[43]

Caution: Although you can buy isoflavone supplements, many experts advise against them since too many soy chemicals can interfere with thyroid action, mineral absorption, or mental function. There's conflicting evidence about whether soy can help or hinder breast cancer, so if you have or have had the disease or have a family history of breast cancer, be very cautious about using soy or soy products. Eating soy or soy products may also trigger allergic reactions or gastrointestinal difficulties. Consult your physician before using soy or soy products to prevent or decrease heart disease.

Recommendation: The FDA says that 25 grams of soy protein daily plus a diet low in saturated fat and cholesterol may lower blood cholesterol and the risk of heart disease. But an analysis of 35 studies on soy found that it takes closer to 47 grams of soy protein per day to achieve a 9 percent drop in total cholesterol and a 13 percent drop in LDL.[44] You can get approximately 25 grams of soy protein by consuming ½ cup roasted soy nuts, 1 oz of soy protein isolate, 10 oz of tofu, 2.5 oz soy flour, or 3 cups of soy milk.

Tea, Black (Camellia sinensis)

Made from the fermented leaves of the *Camellia sinensis* bush, black tea contains flavonoids and other substances that act as antioxidants in the body and can help reduce both total and LDL cholesterol.

- The results of a 1992 Norwegian study of 9,857 men showed that the more black tea the men consumed, the lower their total cholesterol levels and blood pressure. And those who drank one or more cups of tea daily during the 12-year follow-up period had a lower death rate than those who didn't drink tea at all.[45]
- Researchers in Israel found that black tea drinkers had lower total cholesterol levels compared to coffee drinkers, who had higher total cholesterol and higher LDL levels.[46]
- Dutch researchers followed 805 men for 5 years, looking at their intake of flavonoids, most of which came from black tea. The researchers found that the higher the flavonoid intake, the lower the risk of death from heart disease.[47]

Caution: Black tea contains caffeine, so if you're caffeine sensitive, try a decaffeinated variety or drink green tea, which contains about half the caffeine.

Recommendation: Drink 1–2 cups of black tea daily.

Tea, Green (Camellia sinensis)

Popular in Asia for centuries, green tea is made from the unfermented leaves of the *Camellia sinensis* bush (as opposed to the fermented leaves used in black tea). Green tea contains *catechin*, a particularly potent antioxidant from the polyphenol family. Catechin helps protect against heart disease by keeping total cholesterol and LDL down and HDL up, preventing "sticky" platelets from clogging up arteries, and warding off the oxidation of LDL.

- In Japan, a study of 1,306 men found that the more green tea they consumed, the lower their total cholesterol levels. There was an average 8 mg/dL drop in total cholesterol in those who drank 9 or more cups of green tea daily, compared with those who drank 0–2 cups per day, which translates to a 16 percent drop in heart disease risk.[48]
- Green tea was found to lower blood fats and decrease the tendency toward atherosclerosis, especially when intake was greater than 10 cups per day, according to a study of 1,371 men in Yoshimi, Japan.[49]
- Researchers in China found that green tea decreased platelet stickiness, clotting, and the amount of cholesterol deposited on artery walls, and that it could even help break down already-formed blood clots.[50]
- Finally, green tea appears to lower the risk of stroke. Researchers who studied 6,000 Japanese people age 40 and up found that those who drank more than 5 cups of green tea daily had less than half the strokes (whether caused by clots or cerebral hemorrhage) than those who drank fewer cups.[51]

Recommendation: The heart-protective effects of green tea are most evident when at least 3 cups of the tea are consumed daily. If you're not a tea drinker, try taking 240–320 mg of green tea extract in capsule form.

Vitamins and Minerals

Several vitamins and minerals play important roles in general heart health. Others may have direct effects on cholesterol levels.

Carotenoids

Carotenoids are a family of colorful pigments found in plants that have strong antioxidant properties. Of the more than 600 carotenoids identified to date, beta-carotene is the most famous, but other well-known cousins are alpha-carotene, lycopene, lutein, zeaxanthin, and cryptoxanthin. A number of large population studies have linked the carotenoids to the prevention of heart disease:

- A 13-year study of 1,899 men with elevated total cholesterol and blood fats found that the greater the carotenoid levels in their blood, the lower their risk of coronary heart disease.[52]
- A Swiss study divided 2,974 middle-aged men into four groups according to how much carotene was in their blood. Those in the group with the lowest carotene levels were at increased risk of dying of coronary artery disease.[53]
- An 8-year study of more than 87,000 healthy U.S. women divided the subjects into five groups according to the amount of beta-carotene they consumed. Those in the group that consumed the most beta-carotene were 22

percent less likely to suffer from coronary artery disease than those in the group that consumed the least.[54]

You can find carotenoids in yellow, orange, and red fruits and vegetables (e.g., carrots, squash, papaya, cantaloupe, pumpkin, tomatoes, and red peppers), as well as in dark green vegetables like broccoli and spinach. Eat them fresh and raw, not cooked, since cooking can easily deplete the carotenoid content.

Caution: If you have hypothyroidism, you may not be able to convert beta-carotene into vitamin A, so avoid taking beta-carotene supplements.

Recommendation: Eat at least one serving of a beta-carotene-rich food each day. A typical dosage in supplement form is 25,000 IU (15 mg) of beta-carotene daily.

Folic Acid

Named for *folium*, the Latin word for leaf, this member of the B family of vitamins is found in dark green leafy vegetables, brewer's yeast, beets, liver, broccoli, and orange juice. In combination with vitamins B_6 and B_{12}, folic acid helps to control the levels of *homocysteine*, an amino acid that can cause the scratches in blood vessel walls that lead to atherosclerosis. High blood levels of homocysteine have been linked to blood clots, blood vessel disease, and a greater risk of heart attack.[55]

- Postmenopausal women with high levels of homocysteine were able to lower their circulating levels of this amino acid by taking 5 mg folic acid per day for 4 weeks.[56]
- An increase in homocysteine levels caused by

taking the drug fenofibrate was kept at bay by daily doses of 650 mcg of folic acid, 5 mg of B_6 and 50 mcg of B_{12}.[57]

- In a test of folic acid's ability to ward off heart problems, 17 elderly patients suffering from arteriosclerosis (hardening of the arteries) were given between 5 and 7.5 mg of folic acid daily. As a result, capillary blood flow improved.[58]

Caution: Taking too much folic acid may cause rashes, itching, allergic bronchospasms, or fatigue.

Recommendation: Typical doses for healthy people range from 400–800 mcg. However, the best results for those with atherosclerosis or high homocysteine levels have been achieved with doses of 500–750 mcg. Consult your physician before taking more than 800 mcg of folic acid.

Magnesium

This mineral is a sort of jack of all trades when it comes to heart health. Among other things, it helps keep the heart beating properly, reduce total cholesterol, increase HDL, and prevent unnecessary clumping in the blood that can trigger a heart attack.[59] A lack of magnesium can cause irregular heartbeat, high blood pressure, heart failure[60] and sudden heart attacks.[61] On the other hand, getting plenty of magnesium may help prevent the scratches that begin the process of atherosclerosis, ward off future heart attacks, and lower the death rate in those who have already had them.

- In animal studies, magnesium-deficient diets caused lesions (scratches) in the hearts and arteries of all animals studied. When the animals consumed a diet that was high in saturated fat *and* low in magnesium, the lesions were intensified. But taking magnesium supplements helped to prevent the number of lesions.[62]

- A British study involving 2,000 patients followed for a period of 4 years showed that heart attack patients treated with magnesium were 20 percent less likely to die during that period than those who didn't take the mineral.[63]

- In a study involving 2,300 people, some were given magnesium injections while they were in the process of having a heart attack. The injections cut their death rate by 25 percent, as compared to those who didn't get the injections.[64]

Although the jury is still out on just how magnesium prevents future heart attacks, it's believed to widen the coronary arteries, improve blood flow, and stabilize the heart rhythms.

Caution: Large amounts of magnesium supplements can be toxic if taken over time, especially if you have kidney disease or your calcium and phosphorus intakes are high. Don't take more than 3,000 mg of magnesium supplements per day.

Recommendation: Typical doses are about 500 mg magnesium per day, in supplement or food form. Good sources of magnesium include nuts, legumes, whole grains, dark green vegetables, and seafood.

Niacin

A member of the B family of vitamins, niacin has long been known to reduce total cholesterol and LDL, while raising HDL. Although scientists aren't exactly sure why niacin works, it appears to block the manufacture and secretion of LDL.[65] Whatever the reason, high doses of niacin appear to help regulate cholesterol levels.

- Researchers from Duke University Medical Center tested the ability of an extended-release form of niacin to raise low levels of HDL. Niacin was compared to a standard cholesterol-lowering drug in this double-blind study of 173 people. The niacin raised HDL 21–25 percent, depending on the dose, and did a better job raising HDL than the drug.[66]
- A 2000 study published in the *Journal of the American Medical Association* examined the use of niacin in 468 people suffering from peripheral artery disease, including 125 with diabetes. Some participants were given up to 3,000 mg of niacin per day for as long as 60 weeks; others got a placebo. Niacin pushed down LDL by as much as 9 percent, lowered the blood fats by up to 28 percent, and increased the HDL by 29 percent.[67]
- In a study of 29 men and women with ischemic heart disease and elevated cholesterol/blood fats, taking either 1.5 grams or 3.0 grams of niacin significantly lowered the total cholesterol, LDL cholesterol, and blood fats, while raising the HDL.[68]

Caution: Taking large doses of niacin (e.g., 3,000 mg per day) may cause reddening of the face, tingling sensations, itching, nausea, vomiting, diarrhea, dizziness, liver dysfunction, or high blood sugar levels. Do not take niacin if you have liver disease, an active peptic ulcer, severe low blood pressure, or arterial bleeding. Do not take niacin in conjunction with cholesterol-lowering drugs.

Recommendation: In order to lower LDL and triglycerides and raise HDL, high doses of niacin (in the form of nicotinic acid) must be taken. A typical dose to lower cholesterol is up to 1,000 mg, two to three times a day. These high doses should only be used under the watchful supervision of a physician. Liver tests should be performed regularly to ensure that this therapy is not damaging the liver.

Selenium

Selenium is necessary for production of *glutathione peroxidase*, the body's primary antioxidant, which plays a pivotal role in preventing cancer, heart disease, and other conditions.[69] The amount of selenium in the blood and the red blood cells seems to be related to the risk of heart disease and heart attacks;[70] that is, the lower the level of selenium, the greater the risk. This may be because selenium's antioxidant abilities ward off the oxidation of LDL. Selenium also helps thin the blood,[71] making it less likely that unnecessary blood clots will form and trigger a heart attack. Among patients who had heart attacks, those treated with selenium or selenium-rich yeast were less likely to have second attacks than those who were given a placebo.[72]

Caution: Experts recommend against long-term use of more than 200 mcg of selenium a day until it's proven by authorities to be safe. Short-term use of as much as 600 mcg daily may be acceptable for a few days only, but doses of 900 mcg or more can be toxic. Signs of toxicity include nausea, vomiting, a garlicky breath odor, brittle nails, loss of hair, and a metallic taste in the mouth.

Recommendation: Eat selenium-rich foods such as seafood, liver, kidney, wheat germ, onions, and broccoli. In addition, you may wish to take a daily dose of 100–200 mcg of selenium in supplement form.

Vitamin B₆

Vitamin B_6 plays important roles throughout the body as a coenzyme in more than 100 metabolic processes and as a synthesizer of antibodies, brain chemicals, and genetic material. It also helps prevent heart disease, strokes, depression, insomnia, PMS, and several other conditions.[73] In combination with folic acid and vitamin B_{12}, vitamin B_6 helps break down the amino acid homocysteine,[74] which damages artery linings and promotes atherosclerosis. Studies involving animals have shown that diets deficient in B_6 can lead to hardened, narrowed arteries.[75]

Caution: Serious nerve damage can occur when high doses of B_6 (2,000 mg) are taken for more than a few weeks. Numbness and tingling in the hands and feet or poor coordination can result from doses as low as 500 mg. Generally, no more than 100–200 mg of B_6 should be taken without a doctor's supervision. B_6 should not be taken in conjunction with levodopa, a drug taken for Parkinson's disease, as it interferes with the action of the drug.

Recommendation: Typical doses of vitamin B_6 are 50–100 mg a day, although as little as 5 mg per day may help keep homocysteine levels in check. Since the B vitamins work together, take equal amounts of B_6, thiamin, riboflavin, and niacin to prevent deficiencies.

Vitamin B₁₂

Vitamin B_{12} is primarily involved in the metabolism of folic acid, so without enough B_{12}, you can develop a folic acid deficiency. It also plays an important part in nerve function. B_{12} contributes to heart health by working together with folic acid and B_6 to prevent the buildup of homocysteine in the blood.[76] While vegans usually have lower than average cholesterol levels, they also have higher than average homocysteine levels, which is most likely due to their poor B_{12} status. One study found that 78 percent of vegans were deficient in B_{12} as opposed to 9 percent of meat eaters.[77]

Caution: Although there are no reported cases of vitamin B_{12} toxicity, large amounts may cause diarrhea, itching, or swelling. Taking large amounts of vitamin C within an hour of taking B_{12} can destroy the action of the B_{12}.

Recommendation: Concentrated amounts of B_{12} are found only in animal foods (e.g., liver, pork, beef, fish, eggs, and milk), so strict vegans who eat no eggs or dairy products can develop a B_{12} deficiency if they don't take a daily B_{12} supplement of at least 2 mcg. Good results in controlling homocysteine levels have been found at 50 mcg per day, although typical daily dosages range from 5–100 mcg.

Vitamin C

Vitamin C, possibly the best known of all of the vitamins, is a strong antioxidant that also plays a role in the conversion of cholesterol into bile acids. If C is lacking, less cholesterol is converted into bile acids, allowing it to build up in the arteries, blood, and liver. Vitamin C is also needed for the normal metabolism of blood fats, which might otherwise contribute to the blocking of the arteries. It's needed to build collagen, which helps keep artery walls strong. And vitamin C is an antioxidant that helps control LDL oxidation and free radical damage to artery walls. Taking all of this into account, it's easy to see how getting plenty of vitamin C could help prevent cardiovascular disease and lower total cholesterol levels.

- Researchers in the United Kingdom spent 4 years examining the link between blood levels of vitamin C, cardiovascular disease, cancer, and death in 19,496 middle-aged and senior men and women. The study revealed that having more vitamin C in the blood reduced the risk of cardiovascular disease, heart attacks, and deaths from all causes.[78]
- From Japan came a 2002 study that compared the amount of vitamin C in the blood with cholesterol. There was an inverse relationship: that is, the more vitamin C, the less LDL.[79]
- A study published in *Atherosclerosis* in 2001 noted that a lack of vitamin C is associated with damage to artery linings and the development of atherosclerosis. In addition, researchers found that taking vitamin C may prevent or treat atherosclerosis through C's antioxidant, anti-infective, and anti-inflammatory actions.[80]

Caution: High doses of vitamin C can result in diarrhea, cramps, bloating, or excessive urination. It can also increase the risk of kidney stones, produce occult blood in the stool, and interfere with anticlotting medication. Doses greater than 1,000 mg can increase oxidation reactions—meaning they can have the opposite effect of an antioxidant. High doses of vitamin C can also wash away folic acid and vitamin B_{12}, so be sure to get the recommended daily amount of each of these water-soluble vitamins.

Recommendation: Recent studies suggest that daily doses of 500–1,000 mg of vitamin C can raise the HDL while lowering LDL.

Vitamin E
Most of vitamin E's beneficial effect has to do with protecting the body against free radical damage, but

it also helps boost the immune system, promote wound healing, improve circulation, and decrease inflammation. Like vitamin C, vitamin E protects the heart by preventing the oxidation of LDL, and it may increase the protective HDL. It also helps regulate the repair process of cells lining the artery walls, and may protect them from the effects of damaging oxidants.[81] In addition, it thins the blood, decreasing the likelihood of blood clots forming that can trigger a heart attack.

Various studies show that vitamin E is truly heart protective:

- In 2001, Australian researchers published the results of a study looking at the link between antioxidant vitamins and atherosclerosis of the carotid arteries. They studied the diets of 1,111 people, checked their blood levels of antioxidant vitamins, and studied their carotid arteries via ultrasound. The researchers concluded that increasing the dietary intake of vitamin E could decrease the risk of atherosclerosis.[82]
- Italian researchers used ultrasound to detect early signs of atherosclerosis in the carotid arteries of 310 women. They found that the women who consumed the most E and those who had the most E in their blood had the fewest signs of carotid atherosclerosis.[83]
- A large-scale study conducted at Harvard involving more than 87,000 female nurses looked at the link between vitamin E intake and the risk of heart disease. The researchers concluded that vitamin E supplementation is associated with a reduced risk of coronary heart disease in middle-aged women.[84]
- In a study involving 34,386 postmenopausal

women, researchers found that the more vitamin E consumed, the lower the risk of death from heart disease.[85]

Caution: Vitamin E thins the blood, so it should not be taken in conjunction with blood-thinning medications. Those who have high blood pressure should avoid high doses of vitamin E, as it can increase the risk of stroke from a blood vessel rupture. More than 2,000 IU of vitamin E per day can interfere with vitamin A absorption.

Recommendation: Studies have shown that daily dosages of 400–800 IU of vitamin E can reduce LDL oxidation, and daily dosages as high as 1,200 IU may be beneficial. Even though vitamin E is itself an antioxidant, as it's metabolized it will produce a certain amount of free radicals. Therefore, you should always take an antioxidant such as vitamin C along with your vitamin E.

Exercise

The higher your HDL, the more protection you have against heart disease, and one of the best ways to raise your HDL is through regular exercise. You don't need to put in long, exhausting hours at the gym to see some effects—just go for a brisk 30-minute walk every day, or take the stairs instead of the elevator. Every little bit helps.

Chapter Five

The Pressure Is On

Although it doesn't hurt and you could easily have it without knowing it, high blood pressure (also known as *hypertension*) is a serious problem that affects some 58 million Americans, or one out of three adults. In 1999 alone, it was directly responsible for about 43,000 deaths and contributed to more than 220,000 others.[1] Hypertension is the number one cause of stroke and greatly increases your risk of developing heart problems. Compared to those with normal blood pressure, people with uncontrolled hypertension are three times more likely to develop heart disease, six times more likely to develop congestive heart failure, and as much as seven to ten times more likely to have a stroke.[2] Although it's easy to dismiss hypertension as another one of those "male diseases," more than half the women age 55 and older have high blood pressure, and some 90,000 women die of strokes every year.[3]

The Problem

High blood pressure can hurt you in several ways. The force generated by the pounding of the blood against artery walls can damage their linings. This causes or contributes to atherosclerosis (the hardening of the arteries due to plaque buildup). These stiff, narrow arteries can't relax and widen enough to deliver enough nutrients and oxygen to the rest of the body, so the organs and tissues they serve (such as the heart, eyes, and kidneys) weaken and decline. Plus the heart must work harder to force the blood through the plaque-choked arteries. The result is an overworked, weakened heart, organ damage, and clogged arteries that can lead to a heart attack or stroke.

Blood Pressure: The Ebb and Flow

Your blood exerts pressure on the insides of your blood vessels as your heart pumps it through your circulatory system. But the pressure isn't constant; it fluctuates as it moves between the "push" and "relax" phases of the heartbeat. The push happens when your heart contracts and sends freshly oxygenated blood into the aorta, the giant artery where blood begins its journey through the body. The relax phase comes between heartbeats, when there's much less force propelling the blood forward.

Doctors measure your blood pressure during each of these phases, and the result is reported in a fraction and in millimeters of mercury—for example, 120/80 mm Hg. The first number is the *systolic pressure*, the pressure in the system during the push phase. The second is the *diastolic pressure*, the pressure in the system during the relax phase.

Blood Pressure by the Numbers

How do you know if you have hypertension? Here are the numbers, according to the American Heart Association:

- optimal—systolic pressure less than 120, *and* diastolic pressure less than 80
- normal—systolic pressure less than 130, *and* diastolic pressure less than 85
- high normal—systolic pressure 130–139, *or* diastolic pressure 85–89

Above this, we get into elevated blood pressure:

- stage 1 (mildly high)—systolic pressure 140–159, *or* diastolic pressure 90–99
- stage 2 (moderately high)—systolic pressure 160–179, *or* diastolic pressure 100–109
- stage 3 (severely high)—systolic 180 or above, *or* diastolic 110 or above

What Causes High Blood Pressure?

So why does blood pressure creep up from the optimal 120/80 to dangerous levels in so many people? The truth is, 90 percent of the time nobody knows, although diet, obesity, alcohol abuse, lack of exercise, stress, genetics, and psychological factors probably play roles. The kind of high blood pressure that has no apparent cause is called *primary hypertension*. Another kind of hypertension, known as *secondary hypertension*, is produced by certain diseases or conditions such as kidney abnormalities, thyroid dysfunction, tumors, or medications. If you have secondary hypertension, you and your doctor will need to work on controlling or eliminating the underlying condition in order to lower your blood pressure.

Primary hypertension also warrants a doctor's close supervision and may require medication to keep it under control. The good news is that many cases of primary hypertension respond very well to simple dietary and lifestyle changes. In fact, you may be able to control your hypertension using natural methods alone.

What Happens When Your Blood Pressure Gets Too High?

Why is high blood pressure such a big deal? It sounds like your heart and blood vessels could be getting a good workout. Wouldn't that make them stronger?

To understand why high blood pressure is so hard on your body, you'll need to visualize your cardio-vascular system as a pump (the heart) connected to a series of tubes (the blood vessels). It's a closed system, so whatever the pump forces through the tubes eventually comes back again. The tubes that carry the blood away from the heart are the arteries; those that bring blood back again are the veins. Since the arteries bear the brunt of the pressure within the system, it's vital that their walls be strong and stretchy, dilating when the blood is pushed through them and contracting a bit during the relaxation phase.

When there's too much pressure in the system, the blood slams away mercilessly against the artery walls (the *endothelium*). This can cause damage (scratches) on the walls that provide a place for plaque buildup and the formation of pockets of plaque within the wall that can eventually rupture. This process signals the beginning of atherosclerosis (the stiffening of the arteries due to plaque buildup on their inner walls).

And atherosclerosis greatly increases the chance of blockages that can trigger a heart attack or stroke.

Endothelial Dysfunction and Atherosclerosis

High blood pressure can also make the endothelium do things it shouldn't. Surprisingly, the endothelium isn't just a layer of cells that lines the inside of the arteries, but an organ in and of itself. It manufactures and secretes several hormones and substances that help control the blood pressure, the stickiness of the blood, and the inflammation process. It also tells the layer of smooth muscle cells within the artery wall to contract or relax, depending on the body's needs for oxygen and nutrients. This muscular layer squeezes the artery passageway to make it narrower and relaxes it to let it widen.

But if the endothelium gets scratched, it doesn't work properly, a condition called *endothelial dysfunction*. The endothelium starts doing things in a crazy way—setting off inflammation when it's not necessary, making the blood stickier, and telling the muscular walls of the arteries to contract for no reason. This encourages both plaque buildup and the narrowing of the arteries, the two hallmarks of atherosclerosis.

As we age, all of us will develop at least some atherosclerosis, much of it originating after damage is done to the endothelium. But in women the process is worsened by the postmenopausal drop in protective HDL and the increase in total cholesterol and LDL. This makes the development of atherosclerosis even more likely. As a result, the heart has to work extra hard to pump blood through the stiffened, narrowed arteries.

High blood pressure, endothelial dysfunction, and atherosclerosis form a vicious circle: high blood pressure causes endothelial dysfunction, which causes atherosclerosis, which narrows the arteries and chokes them with plaque. And narrowed, clogged arteries push the blood pressure up even higher.

In General, You Want To:

- keep your blood pressure below 120/80
- keep arteries flexible and wide
- decrease the workload on your heart
- protect the endothelium from damage
- ward off atherosclerosis
- keep total cholesterol and LDL low
- keep HDL high
- maintain ideal body weight
- exercise regularly

What You Can Do About It

Diet

Adopt the DASH Diet
You may be able to reduce your high blood pressure simply by changing your diet. A special eating plan called the DASH (Dietary Approaches to Stop Hypertension) diet was developed in 1997 by the National Heart, Lung and Blood Institute as part of a study on the effects of groups of nutrients on high blood pressure.[4] Although lots of studies have been

done of the effects of a single nutrient (e.g., vitamin E) on hypertension, the DASH researchers theorized that nutrients grouped together as they're found in foods might be able to lower blood pressure even more effectively. And they were right. When people with untreated hypertension followed the DASH diet for 8 weeks and kept their sodium intakes to moderate amounts (3,000 mg/day), their blood pressures dropped by an average of 11 mm Hg systolic and 5.5 mm Hg diastolic. This is significant, because each reduction of 1 mm Hg in diastolic blood pressure reduces your risk of heart disease by 3 percent and your risk of stroke by 7 percent. The effects of systolic blood-pressure reduction are even better.

When the DASH dieters' sodium intake was lowered to 1,500 mg/day, the results were even better: a decrease of 11.5 mm Hg systolic and 6.8 mm Hg diastolic. And the more that sodium intake was restricted, the lower went the blood pressure. DASH researchers concluded that the blood-pressure-reducing effects of either diet were *just as good as those seen with antihypertensive medications.*

The DASH diet is really not much different than the Mediterranean-style diet referred to in Chapter 4. It emphasizes fresh fruits, vegetables, whole grains, and monounsaturated fats and limited amounts of lean meats, poultry, and low-fat dairy products. The main differences are the DASH diet restricts sodium and the Mediterranean-style diet allows more fat (in the form of olive oil).

The DASH Diet

Food Group	# of Servings	Serving Size	Suggestions
Cereal, grains, pasta	7–8 per day	1 oz dry cereal, ½ cup cooked cereal, 1 slice bread, or ½ cup cooked rice or pasta	Whole wheat breads, cereals, and pastas with no added sugar or salt
Vegetables	4–5 per day	1 medium, 1 cup raw (chopped), ½ cup cooked, or 6 oz vegetable juice	Vegetables should be eaten raw or lightly cooked, without added salt or fats. Vegetable juice can count for *one serving* per day, as long as it contains no salt.
Fruits	4–5 per day	1 medium, 1 cup raw (chopped), ½ cup canned, ¼ cup dried, or 6 oz juice	Fruits should be eaten raw whenever possible. Canned fruits should have no added sugar or syrup.
Meat, poultry, fish	2 or fewer per day	3 oz cooked	Lean cuts only; trim fat; poultry should be eaten without the skin. Baked, broiled or roasted, not fried.
Dried beans, seeds, nuts	4–5 per week	½ cup cooked beans, 2 T seeds, ⅓ cup nuts, or 3 oz tofu	Nuts or seeds should be unsalted. Avoid canned beans because of high sodium/sugar content.

Dairy	2–3 per day	1 cup nonfat or lowfat milk, buttermilk or yogurt, or 1½ oz nonfat or lowfat cheese (low sodium kind)	Use lowfat or nonfat and low sodium dairy products whenever possible. (Dairy products contain sodium.)
Fats, oils	2–3 per day	1 tsp soft margarine, 1 T lowfat mayonnaise, 1 tsp oil, or 2 T light salad dressing	Use monounsaturated oils (olive or canola oil) whenever possible. Avoid saturated fat.
Sweets	5 per week	1 T sugar, or 1 T jelly or jam	Sweets that are low fat are preferable, such as sugar, honey, syrup, or jelly.
Sodium	1,500–3,000 mg per day	About the amount found in ¾–1½ tsp of salt daily (if no other sodium is consumed through foods)	See section on "Lower Your Sodium Intake," below.

Lower Your Sodium Intake

Sodium consumption doesn't affect everyone's blood pressure, but it will if you happen to be sodium sensitive. That's because when you eat salty foods and your blood levels of sodium rise, your body automatically draws more water into your blood to counterbalance the sodium. This increases your blood volume, which raises your blood pressure.

The average American takes in 6,000–10,000 mg of sodium per day (about 3 to 5 tsp of salt), and some people take in much more. Our physiological needs are much less—about ¼ tsp of salt, or 500 mg of sodium per day. You may be able to see a significant drop in your blood pressure (while still enjoying tasty food) just by cutting down to 2,000–3,000 mg of sodium per day, or 1–1½ tsp.

Easing off the Sodium

- Throw away your salt shaker.
- Don't add salt to foods when you're cooking. *Or* use half the salt you'd normally use, then cut it in half again a week later. Keep cutting back until you've stopped adding salt.
- Try using spices or lemon juice for flavoring instead of salt.
- Avoid soy sauce, broth, meat extract, bouillon, or anything cured or pickled.
- Put the contents of canned foods (e.g., tuna) in a strainer and rinse with water to remove some of the sodium.
- Avoid processed foods. (Most of the salt and sodium that we consume comes from them.)
- Take advantage of the many foods that are reduced in sodium or have no salt added.

In addition, watch out for foods that contain any of the following high sodium ingredients:

Baking powder (sodium aluminum sulfate)
Baking soda (sodium bicarbonate)
Barbeque sauce
Bouillon cubes*
Brine
Buttermilk*
Catsup*
Celery salt
Cereal, instant
Cheese (most)*
Corn chips
Cottage cheese
Crackers*
Disodium phosphate
Fish, canned, smoked, or breaded*
Frozen dinners
Garlic salt
Horseradish, prepared
Lemon-pepper spice
Meat extracts
Meat tenderizer*
Meats, canned, smoked, or cured
Meats, Kosher
Monosodium glutamate (MSG)
Mustard, prepared*
Nuts, salted*
Olives*
Onion salt
Party spreads and dips
Peanut butter*
Pickles*
Popcorn, salted*
Potato chips
Pretzels*
Relish
Rennet tablets
Salad dressings, bottled or dry mix
Sauerkraut
Sausage
Sodium alginate
Sodium benzoate
Sodium hydroxide
Sodium propionate
Sodium saccharin
Sodium sulfite
Soups, canned or dry mix
Soy sauce*
Steak sauce
Teriyaki sauce
Vegetable juice, canned*
Worcestershire sauce

Lose excess weight

In most cases, just dropping some extra weight can bring your blood pressure back down to normal levels. In study after study, weight loss has been found

---

*There may be low-sodium versions of these available.

to be one of the most effective ways to reduce blood pressure significantly in hypertensives who are obese or overweight.[5] But you don't have to lose 50 pounds before you see results; even small amounts of weight loss can make a difference in your blood pressure. In two important studies, the Trials of Hypertension Prevention I and II (TOHP I and II), blood pressure was reduced by 7 mm Hg systolic and 5 mm Hg diastolic after a weight loss of slightly less than 10 pounds![6]

Why Is Weight Loss a Key to Controlling Blood Pressure?

Believe it or not, it takes about a mile of capillaries to nourish just one pound of fat. So even a little extra weight can increase your heart's workload dramatically. And just think of the heavy burden straining your heart if you have 20, 50, or 100 pounds of extra fat waiting to be serviced! On the other hand, think of the decreased workload your heart will have when those extra pounds disappear.

A second reason that weight loss eases high blood pressure has to do with a phenomenon called *insulin resistance*. Your body's main fuel, glucose, floats through the bloodstream on its way to feed hungry cells. But it can't enter those cells without the help of the hormone *insulin*. Insulin acts like a key that unlocks the cell's door so that glucose can enter. But in the overweight, fat can block the cell door, making it impossible to insert the insulin key. So the glucose just sails on by, unable to enter the hungry cells and provide nourishment. In effect, an overweight body becomes resistant to the insulin key.

Insulin resistance is bad for your blood pressure. It encourages your body to retain sodium, increasing blood volume and cranking up your blood pressure.

It also speeds up the process of atherosclerosis, narrowing and stiffening your blood vessels and making them more likely to accumulate plaque. Weight loss, however, decreases insulin resistance, which in turn helps to reduce blood volume, decrease atherosclerosis, and normalize blood pressure.[7]

The Best Way to Lose Weight

Your best bet for losing weight and maintaining great health is (once again) the DASH diet (see page 80) or the Mediterranean-style diet (see page 44). If you're emphasizing lots of fresh fruits, vegetables, and whole grains in your diet and eating smaller amounts of meats, poultry, and fish, with nonfat or low-fat dairy products, your calorie intake should be reduced as a result. But if you're still not losing weight, take a look at your portion sizes and the number of portions you're eating. For weight loss, you might consider a plan like this:

1,600 Calorie DASH Diet

Cereal, grains, pasta	6 servings per day
Vegetables	3–4 servings per day
Fruits	3 servings per day
Meat, poultry, fish	1–2 servings per day
Dried beans, seeds, nuts	3 servings per week
Dairy	2 servings per day
Monounsaturated oils	2–3 servings per day
Sweets	2 per week

Any good weight loss program also includes regular exercise. See the exercise recommendations on page 97, later in this chapter.

Take Care with Caffeine

Most studies of large populations don't show a direct relationship between caffeine consumption and a permanent increase in blood pressure.[8] But drinking just one cup of coffee can temporarily increase your heart rate, stiffen your arteries and drive up your blood pressure—effects that are seen almost immediately. A dose of 250 mg of caffeine (about the amount contained in 2 cups of coffee) consumed by a 150-pound person will drive up that person's blood pressure an average of 5–9 mm Hg systolic and 3–8 mm Hg diastolic, if that person hasn't had any caffeine during the previous 12 hours. This increase in blood pressure usually subsides, however, within 30–60 minutes.[9]

If you're hypertensive (or borderline hypertensive), it's a good idea to stay away from anything that increases your blood pressure, temporarily or permanently. Try to keep your caffeine intake to 100 mg per day or less. Remember that prescription drugs can contain caffeine, too, so read the inserts and consult with your health care provider before taking them.

If you're a hard-core coffee drinker, try mixing decaf with your regular coffee and gradually increasing the proportions until you can make the switch to all-decaf. You can also wean yourself away from caffeine by replacing your coffee with black tea (it has less caffeine), then eventually replacing that with green tea (which has even less caffeine).

Coffee (7.5-oz cup)

Drip	115–175 mg
Percolated	80–135 mg
Instant	65–100 mg
Decaffeinated	3–4 mg

Tea (5-oz cup)

Black, 1 min. brew	20 mg
Black, 3 min. brew	35 mg
Green, 1 min. brew	18 mg
Green, 3 min. brew	27 mg

Soft drinks (12 oz)

Mountain Dew	54 mg
Coca-Cola	45 mg
Diet Coke	45 mg
Dr. Pepper	40 mg
Pepsi Cola	38 mg
7-Up	0 mg

Chocolate and cocoa

Baking chocolate (1 oz)	35 mg
Sweet dark chocolate (1 oz)	5–35 mg
Chocolate chips (¼ cup)	12 mg
Cocoa powder, unsweetened (1 T)	11 mg
Milk chocolate (1 oz)	1–15 mg
Chocolate cake (1 slice)	20–30 mg

Over-the-counter medications (caffeine per standard dose)

Caffedrine (stimulant)	200 mg
Dexatrim (stimulant)	200 mg
NoDoz (stimulant)	200 mg
Vivarin (stimulant)	200 mg
Aqua-Ban (diuretic)	200 mg
Pre-Mens Forte (diuretic)	100 mg
Excedrin (pain relief)	130 mg
Anacin, Empirin, Midol (pain relief)	64 mg

Foods and Phytochemicals

There are lots of foods and food components that can help ease your blood pressure down to healthier levels. But just eating a single food or taking a supplement probably isn't going to do the trick. First try following the DASH diet, losing weight, restricting your sodium, and lowering your caffeine intake. Then, for extra ammunition, consider adding some of the following.

Coenzyme Q10

Also known as CoQ10 or ubiquinone (see section on coenzyme Q10, page 47, in Chapter 4), this enzyme is used in the United States, Europe, and Japan to treat high blood pressure, congestive heart failure, angina, and other conditions. A powerful antioxidant, it's intimately tied to the control of high blood pressure. One study showed that giving 100–225 mg of CoQ10 per day to hypertensive patients led to a large and steady drop in blood pressure, with systolic pressure falling by 15 mm Hg and diastolic by 10 mm Hg, on average.[10] Several other studies show similar results:

- In a 1994 study, 26 hypertensive patients with an average blood pressure reading of 164/98 were given 50 mg of CoQ10 twice a day for 10 weeks. Their average systolic reading fell 11 percent, to 147 mm Hg, while their diastolic dropped 12 percent, to 86 mm Hg.[11]
- In another study, 109 hypertensives were given 225 mg of CoQ10 every day for 4 months. Their average systolic pressure fell from 159 to 147 mm Hg, and their diastolic dropped from 94 to 85 mm Hg. *Approximately half of the volunteers*

were then able to stop using one or more of the antihypertensive drugs they had been taking.[12]

- Eighteen hypertensives were given 100 mg of CoQ10 every day for 10 weeks, then a placebo for 10 weeks. During the time they were taking the CoQ10, the average systolic pressure of the patients dropped from 166 to 156 mm Hg, and their diastolic from 103 to 95 mm Hg.[13]

The blood-pressure-reducing effects of CoQ10 are most evident in people with lower levels of CoQ10 (e.g., the elderly or those with diabetes or atherosclerosis). It takes about 4 weeks for the benefits of CoQ10 to reach their peak. Unfortunately, all of the benefits disappear within 2 weeks after it's discontinued.

Caution: See cautions in the section on coenzyme Q10, page 48, in Chapter 4.

Recommendation: Typical doses of CoQ10 are 50–100 mg, twice a day.

Garlic (Allium sativum)

In addition to its ability to help regulate cholesterol levels (discussed in Chapter 4), this herb can help combat hypertension:

- Forty-seven people with mild hypertension were studied by German researchers in 1990. The patients were given either a garlic preparation called Kwai or a placebo for 12 weeks. Among those taking the garlic preparation, diastolic pressure fell from 102 to 89. Total cholesterol and blood fats also fell.[14]
- In a study reported in the *American Journal of Clinical Nutrition* in 1996, patients were given either an aged garlic extract or a placebo for 6

months. The aged garlic reduced the patients' systolic blood pressure by 5.5 percent—and also lowered the total cholesterol and LDL.[15]

- In a recent population survey of 101 adults, researchers found a link between garlic consumption and blood pressure: those who had lower blood pressures ate more garlic.[16]
- Australian researchers reviewing eight different studies on blood pressure and a garlic preparation concluded that the garlic preparation was helpful in treating mild hypertension.[17]

Recommendation: Add garlic to your food whenever possible, eating up to 3 cloves per day.

Omega-3 Fatty Acids/Fish
Several studies have demonstrated that fish or fish oil can reduce elevated blood pressure, especially at large doses.[18] Other studies bear this out:

- Researchers from Harvard's School of Public Health looked at 31 different omega-3/blood pressure studies. They found that fish oil is definitely related to blood pressure, and that there is a "dose-response effect": the more fish oil ingested (up to a certain extent), the more the blood pressure will fall.[19]
- From Norway came a study involving 78 people with untreated hypertension. They were randomly assigned to receive daily doses of either EPA and DHA (the two major omega-3 fatty acids found in fish) or a placebo. Both forms of the fish oil pushed the systolic blood pressure down 3.8 points and the diastolic 2 points more than the placebo did.[20]
- Australian researchers took a look at the fish-

hypertension link combined with weight loss. Sixty-three overweight hypertensives, all taking medicine, were assigned to one of three groups: one ate a fish meal each day; one ate a fish meal and dieted to lose weight; and one, the control group, followed no special regimen. At the end of the 16-week study period, the researchers found that in the group eating one fish meal per day, systolic pressure fell by 6 points and diastolic by 3. But among those who ate a fish meal every day *and* lost weight, systolic pressure fell by 13 points and diastolic by 9.3.[21]

Caution: See cautions in the omega-3 fatty acids/fish section, page 53, in Chapter 4.

Recommendation: To lower high blood pressure, some experts recommend taking 3–4 grams of omega-3 fatty acids per day.

Soluble Fiber

Soluble fiber is a food fiber that either swells or dissolves in water and is well known for its ability to delay gastric emptying, slow the absorption of glucose into the bloodstream, and lower blood cholesterol. (See section on oat bran, page 51, in Chapter 4.) This kind of fiber helps to lower blood pressure by improving insulin sensitivity, reducing endothelial dysfunction, lowering blood volume, and easing constriction of the blood vessels, among other things.[22] Oats and oat products, the peels of citrus fruits, the skins of beans, guava, psyllium seed, and guar gum are all common sources of soluble fiber that may help control high blood pressure.

- Oat bran given to hypertensive patients reduced their blood pressure an average of 7.5 mm Hg systolic and 5.5 mm Hg diastolic. It took 60 grams of oatmeal, 40 grams of oat bran, or 7 grams of psyllium seed per day to get these results.[23]

- Soluble fibers were also found to reduce the amount of blood pressure medication needed in hypertensive patients.[24]
- Researchers using the soluble fiber glucomannan were able to reduce the systolic blood pressure by 9.4 mm Hg in hypertensive subjects.[25]

Caution: See cautions in the section on oat bran, page 51, in Chapter 4.

Recommendation: A typical daily dose for reducing blood pressure is 60 grams oatmeal, *or* 40 grams oat bran (dry), *or* 3 grams beta glucan, *or* 7 grams psyllium seed.

Vitamin and Minerals

Calcium

Higher amounts of calcium in the diet have been linked to lower blood pressure and a decreased risk of developing hypertension.[26] The link between calcium and blood pressure was brought to the fore in a big way in 1984, when data was analyzed from the first National Health and Nutrition Examination Survey.[27] The analysis showed that people with hypertension were more likely to be taking in low levels of calcium, compared to their intakes of other nutrients.

- In 1997, results of the DASH study were published in the prestigious *New England Journal of Medicine*. This study showed that blood pressure could be lowered by eating a diet rich in fruits and vegetables—and that results could be enhanced by eating three servings daily of dairy products.[28]

- Information from over 55,000 registered nurses in the United States, ages 34–59, was used to calculate the effects of calcium on blood pressure. The study's authors compared the amount of hypertension in women taking 800 or more mg of calcium per day to those consuming less than 400 mg daily. The risk of developing hypertension was significantly less in those taking the larger amount.[29]

- A careful examination of 42 different studies on calcium found a clear and convincing link between calcium and hypertension, and concluded that dietary calcium had a stronger antihypertensive effect than calcium from supplements.[30]

Caution: Lowering blood pressure by using calcium supplements alone, without the use of magnesium supplements, can result in calcium deposits in the kidneys.[31] Calcium supplements may cause gastrointestinal bleeding and distress in some people, and taking large amounts for long periods might increase the risk of prostate cancer and other problems. If you have renal disease, check with your physician before taking calcium. Calcium supplements may interfere with absorption of iron, zinc, and magnesium and may interfere with estrogen, certain antibiotics, and other medications.

Recommendation: In food or supplement form, take in a total of 1,000–1,500 mg of calcium daily, plus half as much magnesium (500–750 mg). Calcium is better absorbed from foods, especially dairy products, than from supplements.

Magnesium

An important component of our bones and teeth, this mineral plays a role in hundreds of metabolic tasks within the body, from protein digestion to the manufacture of insulin. Various studies show that magnesium can also help keep the heart beating properly and the arteries clear.

- Studies of large population groups have shown that there's a reverse relationship between magnesium and blood pressure: more magnesium in the diet equals lower blood pressure, while less magnesium in the diet equals higher blood pressure.[32] In most of these population studies, as well as in clinical trials, 500–1,000 mg of magnesium per day is enough to reduce blood pressure.
- Ninety-one women, middle-aged and older, all suffering from mild to moderate hypertension, were enrolled in a double-blind, placebo-controlled study. Some of them were given 485 mg of magnesium per day, others a placebo. After 6 months of treatment, the average systolic blood pressure fell 2.7 points and the diastolic 3.4 points in those taking the magnesium.[33]
- Information from over 55,000 female nurses was used in a major study looking at the effects of various nutrients on blood pressure. Women taking in 300 mg of magnesium per day or more were significantly less likely to develop hypertension than those who consumed 200 mg or less every day.[34]

Caution: Large amounts of magnesium can be toxic if taken over time, especially if you have kidney disease or your calcium and phosphorus intakes are high. Don't take more than 3,000 mg per day.

Recommendation: 500–1,000 mg per day in food or supplement form.

Potassium

The third most common mineral in the human body, potassium is found mainly inside our cells. We need potassium to make sure that our body fluids are properly distributed, nerve impulses speed through the nervous system, and our muscles contract and relax at the right times. This mineral also helps regulate both heartbeat and blood pressure.

Hypertension experts recommend that we take in about five times as much potassium as sodium, but the average American gets about twice as much sodium as potassium.[35] That's too bad, because a high potassium intake may help relax constricted arteries,[36] as well as reduce the incidence of heart attacks and strokes.[37]

- Many studies have shown that when the amount of potassium in the diet goes up, the blood pressure goes down.[38] Adding 2,400–4,800 mg of potassium per day has been shown to lower systolic pressure by 4.4 points and diastolic by 2.5 points in hypertensive people.[39]
- When 150 Chinese men and women, ranging in age from 35 to 64, were given 2,400 mg of potassium every day for 12 weeks, their systolic pressure fell an average of 5 points. And the higher their blood pressure had been at the beginning of the study, the more they responded to the mineral.[40]

- An analysis of data from the Third National Health and Nutrition Examination Survey showed that potassium was inversely linked to blood pressure.[41] That is, the greater the intake of potassium, the lower the blood pressure.

Caution: Excessive amounts of potassium are usually excreted through the urine, so those with kidney disease should not eat high-potassium foods or take potassium supplements. Doses of 18,000 mg or more can be toxic.

Recommendation: Many experts advise an intake of 2,400 mg of potassium per day in food or supplement form. You can get potassium by eating citrus fruits, bananas, green leafy vegetables, sunflower seeds, and tomatoes.

Vitamin C

While we still may be wondering if vitamin C cures the common cold, there's no doubt that it combats cardiovascular disease, diabetes, and cataracts, while strengthening the immune system. A powerful antioxidant, vitamin C helps to keep the blood vessels in good working order, fights atherosclerosis, improves endothelial dysfunction, and keeps LDL cholesterol levels down.

A large number of studies have linked vitamin C to blood pressure, showing that as dietary or blood levels of vitamin C rise, blood pressure decreases.[42] Conversely, less vitamin C means higher blood pressure. And hypertensives tend to have significantly less vitamin C in their bloodstreams than people with normal blood pressures.[43]

- Twenty-three hypertensive women, with blood pressures ranging from 140/90 to 160/100, were given 1,000 mg vitamin C daily for three months. Their systolic pressure fell by an average of 7 points, their diastolic by 4.[44]

- Thirty-nine volunteers with hypertension were enlisted in a 4-week study. Some were given an initial dose of 2,000 mg vitamin C, followed by 500 mg of vitamin C daily; the others received a placebo. The vitamin reduced the systolic pressure by an average of 11 points, the diastolic by 6.[45]

- Thirty-one people with stage 1 hypertension participated in an 8-month study. They were given either 500 mg, 1,000 mg, or 2,000 mg of vitamin C daily. In all groups, the systolic pressure fell an average of 4.5 points and the diastolic 2.8 points within a month, and remained there for the rest of the 8-month study. There was no additional benefit for a dose higher than 500 mg.[46]

Caution: See cautions in the vitamin C section in Chapter 4, page 70.

Recommendation: Eat plenty of foods containing vitamin C, such as citrus fruits, papayas, guavas, red peppers, cantaloupes, black currants, and sweet green peppers. You may also want to take a 250–500 mg supplement twice a day.

Exercise

Dr. Mark Houston, one of the nation's foremost experts on blood pressure, calls exercise "one of the most powerful non-drug remedies for the prevention and treatment of hypertension."[47] The surgeon general of the United States agrees, stating that people with hypertension can effectively lower their blood pressure just by engaging in moderately intense physical activity such as brisk walking for 30–45 minutes a day, almost every day.[48]

How does it work? Various studies have found that exercise helps you lose weight, decreases arterial resistance to blood flow, improves endothelial function, lowers LDL, raises HDL, reduces formation of blood clots, and improves blood flow to the heart.[49] All of these translate to lower blood pressure and a cardiovascular system that functions on a higher level.

- Twenty-three patients with mild hypertension were enrolled in a study testing the effects of moderately intense exercise. Twelve weeks later, systolic blood pressure had fallen an average of 18 points in those who had exercised. Their total cholesterol and LDL had also dropped, while their HDL had risen.[50]

- A study published in the *American Journal of Hypertension* focused on 42 men and women with "white coat hypertension" (the tendency of blood pressure to rise when it's being measured by a health professional). Half of the participants exercised three times weekly; the others did nothing special. After only 4 weeks, the exercise group showed significant decreases in blood pressure, total cholesterol, LDL, and triglycerides and elevations in HDL, results that were maintained throughout the course of the 12-week study. At study's end, the average decrease in blood pressure was 11 points systolic and 5 points diastolic.[51]

- A review of 54 different studies investigated the relationship between exercise and hypertension. This analysis found that aerobic exercise could, on average, lower systolic pressure by 3.8 points and diastolic by 2.7.[52]

Although you might think that all that physical activity would make your blood pressure rise, the overall effect is just the opposite. Because once you've finished your exercise session, your blood pressure can drop to a lower level than before you exercised, and stay there for hours! A study of mildly hypertensive men engaging in physical activity found a drop in blood pressure that lasted 8–12 hours after they finished exercising. Also, their blood pressure was lower on exercise days than on non-exercise days.[53]

Caution: Be sure to consult with your physician when you start a new exercise regimen or add to your current program. Work with a qualified physical therapist or exercise therapist to make sure you're doing every exercise and activity the right way, that you're properly dressed and equipped, and that you're doing only as much as your body can comfortably handle.

Recommendation: For maximum cardiovascular benefits, perform aerobic exercise, the kind that gets your heart beating faster, for 15–30 minutes, 3–5 times a week. Rapid walking, swimming, bicycling, jogging, jumping rope, and sports that require constant fast movement are all forms of aerobic exercise. But your exercise program doesn't have to be exhausting to be productive. Researchers from the University of Tennessee found that among postmenopausal women with borderline or mild hypertension, those who simply walked two miles a day could lower their systolic blood pressure by a whopping 11 points.[54]

Lifestyle Changes

Stop Smoking

Every smoker is at risk of developing heart disease, particularly if she has high blood pressure or high cholesterol levels. The nicotine in cigarettes increases the heart rate, and increased levels of carbon monoxide in the blood squeeze out the oxygen, forcing the heart to work doubly hard. At the same time, smoking causes the blood vessels to constrict, making it more difficult to pump the blood through them.

Cigarette smoke is loaded with free radicals that injure blood vessel linings, contribute to the oxidation of LDL, and eat up your precious antioxidants. Is it any wonder that smokers have a high incidence of atherosclerosis? Women who smoke and take birth control pills are really rolling the dice: they have 22 times the risk of suffering a heart attack compared to nonsmokers.[55]

Recommendation: Stop smoking cigarettes, cigars, and pipes. Completely. Now. You may want to consult with your doctor as to how to use nicotine patches or gum, where to find a support group, or how to use other self-help techniques.

Cut Back on Alcohol Intake

Heavy drinking of alcoholic beverages will definitely drive up your blood pressure[56] and contribute mightily to your chances of having a stroke.[57] Although initially alcohol widens your blood vessels, your body will soon respond by constricting them, pushing your blood pressure way up.

Having more than about two drinks a day (20 grams of alcohol) will increase both your risk of developing hypertension and its severity. It will also interfere with the action of any blood pressure-lowering medications. And even if you don't have hypertension and have no risk factors for it, you stand a good chance of developing high blood pressure if you drink more than about 16 beers per week (210 grams of alcohol).[58]

Recommendation: If you drink, do so in moderation, which means less than 10 oz of wine, *or* 24 oz of beer, *or* 2 oz of hard liquor per day.

Manage Stress

During stressful times, your sympathetic nervous system leaps into action, flooding your body with powerful stress chemicals that can put a strain on your heart, cause endothelial dysfunction, promote atherosclerosis, and otherwise ratchet up your blood pressure.

Numerous studies have implicated stress as a contributor to hypertension. For example, in a study reported in *Psychophysiology* in 2001, researchers at UCLA looked at 203 healthy female registered nurses who rated their moods many times a day.[59] The monitoring of their blood pressure revealed that when the women's "negativity" rose, so did their blood pressure. In a different study, the same researchers found that among male and female college students, sad feelings were linked to elevations in blood pressure and pleasant feelings to drops in blood pressure.[60]

Fortunately, numerous studies have shown that stress management can help bring elevated blood pressure back down. Whether in the form of cognitive therapy, relaxation, meditation, biofeedback, autogenic training, or progressive relaxation, stress management can be quite helpful.

- A recent review of studies testing the effects of a form of self-relaxation called autogenic training looked at more than 30 different controlled trials. The researchers found this form of stress management helpful in treating mild-to-moderate hypertension, as well several other disorders.[61]
- Cognitive behavioral therapy was put to the test in a group of patients who were given medications for their hypertension. The key finding was that a year later, those who had been given the therapy were far less likely to require blood pressure medication, compared to those who had not had the therapy.[62]
- Researchers from the University of South Florida looked at the effects of stress management in African-American women, who are known to be at high risk of developing hypertension. Some of the women in the study were asked to practice progressive relaxation, the others to simply relax for 30 minutes a day. In the progressive relaxation group, the average systolic blood pressure fell from 130 to 121 mm Hg, while the other group showed no change.[63]

Recommendation: Shed all the stress you can. Try aromatherapy, autogenic training, biofeedback, cognitive behavioral therapy, deep breathing, meditation, prayer, progressive relaxation, qi gong, relaxation tapes, self-hypnosis, soothing music, tai chi, warm baths, yoga, or whatever it takes to keep your cool.

Rising Stars?

Here are some substances that may, when more research with human subjects is conducted, prove to be valuable.

- *Hawthorn*—A traditional remedy for heart disease, this herb has mild, positive effects on hypertension, although they can take several weeks to be felt.[64]
- *L-arginine*—This amino acid is a precursor to nitric oxide, which the body uses to keep blood vessels wide open and blood pressure under control. A small study in which participants were asked to eat different types of diets showed that adding L-arginine to the diet could lower blood pressure.[65]
- *Olive leaf*—Extract of the olive leaf contains phytochemicals that, among other things, may encourage the arteries to dilate, thus helping to combat elevated blood pressure. In one study, taking an olive leaf extract for 3 months led to a statistically significant drop in blood pressure.[66]
- *Red clover*—A study of the effects of a red clover extract called Promensil in 17 people found that it improved the flexibility of the arteries and could thus be helpful in treating hypertension.[67]
- *Taurine*—This amino acid was put to the test in a study of 19 people with borderline hypertension. Those who were given 6 grams of taurine daily for a week saw their systolic blood pressures drop by an average of 9 points and their diastolic by 4.[68]
- *Yarrow* (Achillea wilhelmsii)—A popular remedy for fevers, this herb was given to 120 men and women suffering from elevated blood pressure or cholesterol. After 6 months of daily treatment, blood pressure dropped significantly.[69]

Chapter Six

Hold On to Your Bones!

If you're over 50, chances are greater than fifty-fifty that you'll develop either low bone mass or *osteoporosis*, a disease that causes bones to become thin, fragile, and easily broken. Of the 44 million Americans who suffer from osteoporosis, some 70 percent are women. How did women get so lucky? To begin with, our bones are smaller, thinner, and less dense than men's. Add to that the hormone changes that speed up bone loss after menopause and the fact that women typically get about half the calcium they need, and the sorry result is *half of all American women over the age of 50 will have an osteoporosis-related fracture at some time during their lives.*[1] Of these women, one-third will have serious bone deterioration, a figure that soars to nine out of ten after age 75.[2]

Right now there are about 28 million women suffering from osteoporosis and low bone mass, resulting in about 1.5 million bone fractures a year.[3] Wrists or forearms may snap while breaking a fall. Vertebrae in the spine can collapse while simply holding up the weight of the body, causing chronic back pain, a curved spine, and a marked loss in height. But possibly worst of all is the broken hip, a phenomenon that sends up to 50 percent of its victims to nursing homes, requires surgery, and causes prolonged disability. Broken hips are particularly scary when you realize that some 20 percent of the elderly who break their hips *end up dying within a year*, usually due to fracture complications.[4] It's estimated that one in seven women will experience a hip fracture during her lifetime, and one in four of these women may die within a year due to complications.[5] To make matters worse, studies of large populations reveal that people with osteoporosis have a significantly greater chance of dying of heart disease and stroke than others of the same age who don't have thinning bones.[6] As a significant cause of disability and possible mortality, osteoporosis is a major health problem.

The Problem

Osteoporosis causes a decrease in bone mass and density that leaves the bones weak, thin, porous, and easily fractured. A major cause of disability, osteoporosis can also be an indirect cause of death. Postmenopausal women are particularly at risk of developing the disease, since a drop in female hormones accelerates bone loss.

If you're like most people, you probably take your bones for granted. They're just there—holding you up and carrying you effortlessly through the thousands of movements you make each day. You may not even realize that they're made up of living, ever-changing tissue, just as your skin, hair, and nails are. Yet special cells are constantly churning out new bone tissue while other cells break down old bone tissue and recycle the minerals it contains.

During your youth (up until you're about 25), the activity of your bone building cells outstripped the activity of your bone breakdown cells, so your bone mass increased. Then, somewhere around age 25, these build-up processes began to slow, producing only small increases during the next few years. Then, once you hit 35, the breakdown of your bones started to exceed the buildup, and your overall bone mass began to decline at the rate of about 1 percent a year. But when you reach menopause and your estrogen levels drop, your bone loss will speed up dramatically for the first 3–5 years, to 2–3 percent a year. Then you'll continue to lose bone for the rest of your life, although the rate of loss will slow, to 1–1.5 percent a year. While 1 or 2 percent may not sound like a lot, when it happens year after year, you can suffer significant bone deterioration. Some women lose as much as 20 percent of their bone density during the 5–7 years following menopause. Add to that a 1.5 percent bone loss each year, and you could wind up with only about 50 percent of your original bone mass by the time you reach age 75!

Who's Most Likely to Get Osteoporosis?

Like most diseases, osteoporosis has its favorite targets. The factors that contribute to osteoporosis risk include:

- being female
- Caucasian or Asian heritage
- slim build, small frame

- inadequate intake of calcium, vitamin D, and vitamin K
- long-term intake of too much vitamin D or vitamin A
- a family history of osteoporosis
- bed rest for a period of months or longer
- excessive intake of wheat bran, sodium, caffeine, phosphorus, or protein
- cigarette smoking
- irregular menstruation
- premature menopause
- estrogen deficiency
- anorexia nervosa
- long-term use of certain medications, including corticosteroids, anticonvulsants, diuretics, antacids, and sleeping pills

The Estrogen-Bone Connection

The standard medical approach to preventing and treating osteoporosis is to use medications that inhibit bone breakdown and maintain bone mineral density. Until recently, estrogen was the drug of choice. Not only does it help slow bone breakdown and prevent fractures of the hip, spine, and other sites,[7] it also plays an indirect part in bone building:

- Estrogen "turns on" the vitamin D receptors in your intestines, so that vitamin D can be absorbed and do its work. Once inside, vitamin D is converted into a hormone that helps your body absorb calcium and phosphorus and deposit them into your bones. The vitamin D hormone also reduces the excretion of calcium through the kidneys, saving it and sending it back into circulation. Too little estrogen can cause a lack of vitamin D activity, making it harder for your body to absorb and retain calcium, so bones weaken, become porous, and break easily.

- Estrogen has a direct connection to bone tissue, which is clearly seen by the presence of estrogen receptor sites on both bone building cells (*osteoblasts*) and bone breakdown cells (*osteoclasts*). Although researchers still don't know exactly how estrogen affects the bone once it connects with these cells, the current theory is that estrogen prolongs the life of the building cells while speeding the death of the breakdown cells.[8] Thus, more bone building and less bone dismantling.

But estrogen isn't a magic pill, by any means. Estrogen replacement works best as a preserver of bone during the first 3–5 years after menopause, when bone breakdown soars. But it doesn't actually build new bone or replace bone that is already lost. And the longer estrogen is used, the less effective it becomes at preventing hip and spinal fractures.[9]

Yet all of this may be a moot point now that using estrogen as a preventive strategy for osteoporosis has to be weighed against its substantial risks for assisting cardiovascular disease and breast cancer. Most women and their health care providers are looking for nonestrogen answers to osteoporosis. And luckily there are plenty of them.

In General, You Want To:

- promote bone buildup
- slow the rate of bone breakdown
- maintain or increase bone density

What You Can Do About It

Diet

Ideally, the prevention of osteoporosis should begin in childhood, when your body is building bone fast and furiously. Getting plenty of calcium and vitamin D at this time is essential in order to build your bones to their maximum density, so that once you start to lose bone tissue, you'll have more to spare. But no matter what your age, diet is vitally important to the health of your bones. In general, consuming a diet rich in fruits, vegetables, and whole grains, such as the Mediterranean-style diet (see Chapter 4, page 44) or the DASH diet (see Chapter 5, page 80), can help. These diets contain plenty of vitamins and minerals essential to bone health, including magnesium, potassium, zinc, boron, vitamin K, and others. You should also pay particular attention to the following:

Get Plenty of Calcium

The mineral calcium is essential to bone building and maintenance. Of the 2–5 pounds of calcium found in our bodies, about 98 percent resides in our bones.[10] Every 7 years our bones completely replace themselves, so a steady supply of calcium is crucial to bone health. Since bone tissue is in a constant state of turnover, its makeup will reflect not only your diet, but your exercise habits, medication intake, hormonal state, genetics, and lifestyle at any given time.

Your bones also act as a sort of "calcium bank," allowing your body to deposit and withdraw at will. Calcium is used for lots of things other than bone health, including blood clotting, muscle contraction, nerve transmission, and cellular metabolism. If you don't take in enough dietary calcium to meet your body's needs, your body will simply take what it wants from your bones. And if this happens often enough, you can wind up with serious bone loss.

But osteoporosis isn't simply a calcium-deficiency disease. Lots of women take in plenty of calcium and still develop osteoporosis. Osteoporosis is a disease characterized by the *loss* of calcium in the bones, and that can be caused by many factors, including diet, vitamin or mineral imbalances, lack of weight-bearing exercise, or hormonal deficiencies, to name a few. So just increasing your calcium intake probably won't be the sole answer to the problem.

For more information on increasing your dietary calcium, see the sections on calcium in "Foods and Phytochemicals" and in "Vitamins and Minerals" later in this chapter.

Watch Your Phosphorus Intake

High amounts of the mineral phosphorus are found in red meat, fish, poultry, carbonated beverages like soft drinks and mineral water, and processed foods containing phosphates. Calcium is best absorbed when there's a calcium-to-phosphorus ratio of 1:1, but most of us are getting more than twice the recommended daily amount of phosphorus (800 mg per day for women 25 or older). While the average American woman takes in well under 800 mg of calcium per day, she also consumes 900–1,700 mg of phosphorus.[11] This is especially true of those of us who substitute soft drinks for milk. Diets that are chronically high in phosphorus and low in calcium are known to speed up bone loss.[12]

Recommendation: Don't overdo it on animal protein. Limit your intake of red meat to one 3-oz serving per week and your carbonated beverage intake to one per day. Don't take vitamin-mineral supplements that have phosphorus added—you're probably getting too much already.

Be Careful with Protein

While adequate protein intake is essential to bone health, too much animal protein increases urinary excretion of calcium and can lead to osteoporosis.[13] Since animal proteins tend to be rich in the highly acidic sulfur-containing amino acids, a buffer is needed to neutralize them, and calcium gets the job. The more animal protein consumed, the more calcium is leached from the bones to buffer its effects. In fact, for every 1 gram increase of protein above the recommended levels, there's a 1.5 gram loss of calcium.[14] Osteoporosis is most prevalent in the areas of the world where a high-protein diet is consumed, particularly if the diet is also low in calcium.

Recommendation: Stick with the RDA of about 50 grams of protein per day (1 oz meat, fish, or poultry = 9 grams; 1 cup milk = 8 grams; 1 cup cooked dried peas or beans = 16 grams). The average American woman consumes about 65 grams of protein daily, 15 grams more than she needs.

Be Careful with Calcium Binders

Certain foods bind up calcium, making it impossible for the body to absorb it. Two of the most notorious are fiber and phytic acid, high amounts of which are found in wheat bran. High fiber diets (those containing more than 35 grams of fiber per day) contribute to osteoporosis, especially if calcium intake is low. Another calcium binder is oxalic acid, which is found in spinach, Swiss chard, beet greens, and rhubarb. But while fiber and phytic acid will bind up the calcium from other foods during the digestion process, oxalic acid simply binds up the calcium found in the same food, so it shouldn't interfere with your absorption of calcium from other foods.

Recommendation: Keep your fiber consumption at or below about 35 grams per day. Don't eat your calcium-containing foods or take calcium supplements at the same time that you eat a high-fiber meal, particularly if the meal contains wheat bran.

Scale Back on Sodium

Taking in too much sodium will increase the amount of calcium you excrete through the urine. A study of Japanese women age 50–79 found that those with a higher sodium intake lost higher amounts of bone breakdown products through the urine.[15] And experts estimate that for every 100 mg of salt you consume, you'll lose 1 mg of calcium.[16]

Recommendation: Keep your sodium intake at or below 3,000 mg per day. (See the "Lower Your Sodium Intake" section in Chapter 5, page 81.)

Curb the Caffeine

Like sodium, caffeine increases the loss of calcium through the urine, and a heavy intake of caffeine will increase your risk of hip fracture.[17] One study found that women who took in the greatest amounts of caffeine (above the 80th percentile) had almost three times as many hip fractures as those who took in the least caffeine.[18] Another study found that women who consumed 1½ times the average amount of caffeine lowered the amount of calcium retained in their bodies by 6 mg/day.[19] The loss of that much calcium on a daily basis could really wallop your bones over time!

Recommendation: Try to keep your caffeine intake to about 100 mg per day, and don't drink soda in place of milk! When you eat or drink something with caffeine, get some calcium at the same time (in food or supplement form) to help stave off caffeine's calcium-robbing tendencies (e.g., put some milk in your coffee). For more information, see "Take Care with Caffeine" in Chapter 5, page 86.

Don't Take Too Much Vitamin A or Vitamin D

Excessive amounts of vitamin A can cause bone abnormalities, increase pain in the bones and joints, and interfere with bone growth. Data from the Nurses' Health Study involving 72,337 postmenopausal women revealed that those taking in the greatest amounts of vitamin A (15,000 IU or more per day) had significantly higher rates of hip fracture than those taking the lowest amounts (less than 6,250 IU per day). Those who took a vitamin A supplement had a 40 percent increased risk of hip fracture, compared to those not taking the supplement. Even those who took in high amounts of vitamin A through food showed an increased risk of hip fracture. But the plant form of vitamin A, beta-carotene, did not contribute to hip fracture.[20]

While you need a certain amount of vitamin D to help absorb calcium, taking too much (more than 1,000 IU) over time can result in calcium deposits in the kidneys and other organs. (See cautions in vitamin D section, page 122.)

Foods and Phytochemicals

Calcium-Rich Foods

As a first line of defense against osteoporosis, the National Institutes of Health recommends the following daily intake of calcium for women:

- 1,000 mg for all women age 25–50

- 1,000–1,500 mg for postmenopausal women under age 65
- 1,500 mg for women over age 65

But most women get about half the recommended amount! And many mistakenly believe that just swallowing a calcium pill will keep osteoporosis at bay and ensure the health of their bones. But more than *half* of the calcium you ingest in supplement form may go unabsorbed. Luckily, the calcium found in foods is much better absorbed, particularly the calcium in dairy products, which come with their very own absorption enhancers, vitamin D and lactose.

Good Sources of Calcium[21]

Food	Serving Size	Calcium per Serving
Dairy Products		
Milk	1 cup	296 mg
Yogurt	1 cup	294 mg
Pudding	1 cup	250 mg
Ice cream	1 cup	236 mg
Cottage cheese	1 cup	230 mg
Cheddar cheese	1 oz	213 mg
American cheese	1 oz	198 mg
Vegetables		
Collard greens	1 cup (cooked)	350 mg
Soybeans, green	1 cup (cooked)	260 mg
Turnip greens	1 cup (cooked)	200 mg
White beans	1 cup (cooked)	200 mg
Chinese cabbage	1 cup (cooked)	150 mg
Mustard greens	1 cup (cooked)	125 mg
Kale	1 cup (cooked)	100 mg
Broccoli	1 cup (cooked)	75 mg

Food	Serving Size	Calcium per Serving
Other		
Sardines (with bones)	3 oz	275 mg
Tofu	4 oz	215 mg
Salmon (with bones)	3 oz	180 mg

Recommendation: Try to get most (if not all) of your daily calcium allotment in food form, if possible. Then add supplements, if necessary. (Also see the section on calcium in "Vitamins and Minerals," page 118.)

Soy or Soybeans

Soy contains *phytoestrogens* (literally, "plant estrogens"), which have mild estrogenlike effects on the body. (See section on "Soy or Soybeans" in Chapter 4, page 58.) Since we know that estrogen preserves bone by protecting it from excessive breakdown, it should be no surprise to learn that the phytoestrogens have the same general effect. Japanese researchers studying postmenopausal women found that those who ate more soy had denser bones than those who ate less.[22]

The phytoestrogens in soy come in the form of *isoflavones*, which are found in nutritionally significant amounts only in soy.[23] Consuming plenty of isoflavones has been linked with better bone density, primarily through protection against bone loss. The traditional Japanese diet contains as much as 150 mg of soy isoflavones per day,[24] while the average American diet contains a measly 1–3 mg. This may be why Japanese women have fewer bone fractures than Western women even though Japanese women don't consume nearly as much calcium and are much less likely to use hormone replacement therapy.

Soy may also help fight osteoporosis by increasing the intestinal absorption of calcium[25] and acting as a source of calcium itself (one 4-oz serving of tofu = 215 mg calcium).

- Chinese researchers gathered together 357 post-menopausal women, recorded their dietary intake of isoflavones, then measured their bone mineral density in two spots. They found that the postmenopausal women who routinely consumed the most dietary isoflavones had better bone mineral densities in the spine and hip.[26]
- A 2002 review article found that when high-isoflavone soy protein was used as an alternative to animal protein in the diet, bone loss in the lumbar spines of peri- and postmenopausal women was inhibited.[27]
- A 24-week double-blind, randomized, placebo-controlled trial of the effect of isoflavones on 69 perimenopausal women used three types of protein: an isoflavone-rich (80 mg) soy protein, an isoflavone-poor (4.4 mg) soy protein, and a protein that contained no isoflavones (whey). While bone densities dropped significantly in the whey group, the isoflavone-rich diet slowed bone loss from the lumbar spine.[28]

A few studies have indicated that isoflavones can also aid in the building of bone:

- In test tube experiments, daidzein (a type of isoflavone) stimulated the proliferation and differentiation of osteoblasts (bone build-up cells), good indications of bone formation.[29]
- In a controlled study, postmenopausal women were given soy protein containing either a

higher or lower amount of isoflavones. Six months later, the women taking the soy with the higher amount (90 mg/day) had significant increases in bone mineral content and bone density in their spines. The women taking the soy with the lower amount did not.[30]

Isoflavones in Foods

This list will give you some idea of which foods contain the most concentrated amounts of isoflavones, but keep in mind that isoflavone content varies from one kind of soybean to the next, as well as from one crop to the next.

Food	Serving Size	Isoflavone Content
Miso	1 T	15 mg
Soy flour	½ cup	50 mg
Soy milk	1 cup	40 mg
Soy nuts, roasted	½ cup	120 mg
Soybeans	1 cup (cooked)	300 mg
Tempeh	½ cup	35 mg
Textured soy protein	¼ cup	60 mg
Tofu	½ cup	35 mg

There is some evidence that fermented soy products such as miso and tempeh are better absorbed than nonfermented soy products. Tofu and soy milk may not be good sources of isoflavones if alcohol processing is used in the manufacturing process.

Caution: There's conflicting evidence about whether soy can help or hinder breast cancer, so if you have (or have had) the disease, or if you have a family history of breast cancer, be very cautious about using soy or soy products. Eating soy or soy products may also trigger allergic reactions or gastrointestinal difficulties. Consult your physician before using soy or soy products to prevent or decrease osteoporosis.

Recommendation: The results of a limited number of human studies on soy and bone health indicate that a daily dose of 50–90 mg of isoflavones is needed before benefits are seen.[31] Although you can buy isoflavone supplements, many experts advise against them since too many soy chemicals can interfere with thyroid action, mineral absorption, or mental function. It's better to get your isoflavones through foods.

Vitamins and Minerals

Although most people think that calcium, by itself, is the answer to osteoporosis prevention, your bones actually need a combination of vitamins and minerals to achieve bone health. They work together in concert, opposing and complementing each other, to achieve a delicate balance that results in strong, healthy bones. Too much or too little of any of these vitamins or minerals can spell disaster for your bones. I've listed the most important contributors to bone health, although there are others that play roles, as well.

Calcium

Calcium carbonate is the cheapest form and provides the most calcium per tablet, but you'll need to have plenty of gastric acid to absorb it properly. As you get older, your production of stomach acid wanes, so you may want to try calcium citrate instead. It contains acid, so it's easier to absorb, although it's also more expensive and you'll have to take either more pills or larger ones. One study pitting calcium carbonate against calcium citrate found that calcium citrate was 2.5 times better absorbed (when taken with meals), and produced a higher peak concentration of calcium in the blood.[32]

Caution: Large doses of calcium can interfere with the absorption of iron, zinc, and other nutrients and may induce constipation and kidney stones. Keep your calcium intake below 2,500 mg per day, particularly if you take it all in supplement form. Calcium-fortified orange juice, cereals, and breads can be used to contribute to calcium intake, but they should be considered supplements, not food sources of calcium.

Recommendation: In the best of all worlds, you'd get your entire calcium allotment from food. If that's unrealistic, try to get at least 600 mg of calcium in food form (e.g., 2 cups milk), then add a supplement to make up the difference. (See sections on calcium in the "Diet" and "Foods and Phytochemicals" sections on pages 109 and 113, respectively.)

Magnesium

An important component of our bones and teeth, magnesium is found in a wide variety of foods, including dark green leafy vegetables, whole-grain breads, nuts, peas and beans. It's necessary for normal growth and maintenance of bone, and works with calcium in both opposing and complementary roles. Since each of these minerals balances the actions of the other, too much or too little of either isn't good for bone health.

Magnesium deficiency is common in women who have osteoporosis and can result in poor bone calcification.[33] The standard American diet is low in magnesium, and magnesium stores can be depleted through alcoholism, chronic diarrhea or vomiting, excessive sugar intake, or the use of certain diuretics. Taking in low amounts of magnesium over a period of just 3 months lowers blood levels of not only magnesium, but also calcium and potassium, so it's important to get good amounts of this mineral in the diet.

- Bone mineral density is directly associated with magnesium intake. A study of women ages 23–75 found that their magnesium intake was a good predictor of the bone mineral content of their forearms.[34]
- In a study of 31 women taking 250–750 mg of magnesium daily for 2 years, almost 75 percent of them enjoyed increases in bone density of 1 to 8 percent. Seventeen other women, who took no supplements, lost between 1 and 3 percent of their bone density during the same period.[35]
- Researchers in Israel found that patients with osteoporosis commonly have magnesium deficiencies, and the magnesium content of their bones is often below normal.[36]

Caution: Taking large amounts of magnesium over time can be toxic, especially if you have kidney disease or your calcium and phosphorus intakes are high. Don't take more than 3,000 mg of magnesium per day.

Recommendation: Intakes of calcium, phosphorus, and magnesium need to be balanced: Keep your total calcium and phosphorus intake about equal, and your total magnesium intake at about half of that (i.e., 1,500 mg calcium, 1,500 mg phosphorus, and 750 mg magnesium). (See "Watch Your Phosphorus Intake," page 110.)

Vitamin D

Vitamin D is essential for adequate absorption of calcium from the intestines and deposition of the mineral into your bones. Vitamin D also salvages calcium that would otherwise be excreted, so your body won't have to draw on the bones to replace it. If you don't have enough vitamin D, you can develop osteoporosis or osteomalacia (literally, "soft bones").

In the United States, milk is typically fortified with vitamin D, but vitamin D deficiencies are becoming more prevalent.[37] This may be because people are getting less exposure to the sun, which is our primary source of this vitamin. When the skin is exposed to the sun's ultraviolet rays, cholesterol within it is converted to vitamin D, a process that takes only about 20 minutes per day of exposure of an area about as big as the back of your hand. Older women, and especially those who live in northern climates, are particularly at risk of vitamin D deficiency because they tend to get outdoors infrequently. This means they must get their vitamin D supply primarily from foods, a less efficient way to go. A study of Muslim women who got little to no sunlight exposure because they were completely veiled found that they had vitamin D deficiencies even when taking 600 IU per day, which is 1½ times the RDA.[38]

Vitamin D deficiencies are also more likely in older women because vitamin D receptors in the gut are estrogen dependent. After menopause, these receptors simply don't absorb vitamin D as well as they used to. Thus, even if a postmenopausal woman is getting plenty of vitamin D in her diet, she could be deficient in vitamin D.

Caution: Over time, taking too much vitamin D in supplement form (more than 1,000 IU per day) can cause calcium deposits in the kidneys and other organs, metabolic disturbances, weakness, diarrhea, mental confusion, and increased urine output. Make sure that you're not doubling up on your intake by taking both a multivitamin *and* a calcium supplement that contain vitamin D, or by taking either supplement along with vitamin D–fortified dairy products.

Recommendation: The National Osteoporosis Foundation recommends a daily dietary intake of 400–800 IU of vitamin D daily. Food sources include fortified dairy products, eggs yolks, and cod liver oil. Getting out in the sun for 20 minutes per day (without sunscreen) may be enough for some people, but others may need food or supplement sources of the vitamin as well.

Vitamin K

Vitamin K is necessary for the manufacture of proteins used in blood clotting, and people who don't get enough of this vitamin tend to bleed excessively and bruise easily. But it's just as important to the maintenance of healthy bones. Vitamin K is needed for the production of a protein found in the bones called *osteocalcin*, which attracts calcium to the bone tissue, where it hardens and crystallizes. Without enough vitamin K, bones can't be built, remodeled, or repaired properly.[39]

In the past, experts believed that it was practically impossible to develop a vitamin K deficiency, since it's found in many plant foods (particularly leafy green vegetables) and manufactured by the intestinal bacteria. But a lack of vitamin K can occur through prolonged use of antibiotics, which destroy many of the friendly intestinal bacteria, or in cases of severe, chronic fat malabsorption.

Recently, scientists have found ways to measure blood levels of vitamin K with greater accuracy than ever before, so they can look at the effects of more subtle drops in vitamin K status. They discovered that lower levels of vitamin K increase the excretion of calcium through the urine.[40] They also found that osteoporosis may be associated with low levels of vitamin K,[41] and that administering vitamin K in these cases reduced urinary calcium loss[42] and helped increase the attraction of calcium to bone tissue (bone building).[43] The current theory holds that too little vitamin K may speed bone loss and interfere with bone building, resulting in osteoporosis.

- An analysis of the results of the Nurses' Health Study, which involved 72,337 postmenopausal women, found that women who consumed greater amounts of vitamin K had fewer hip fractures.[44]
- Dutch researchers studied the capacity of osteocalcin, the bone protein, to attract calcium (an indirect measurement of bone-building ability) in 50 healthy postmenopausal women age 55–75. Their osteocalcin had less than half the normal calcium-attracting capacity. But after just 2 weeks of vitamin K therapy at 1 mg/day, osteocalcin/calcium activity was back to normal, suggesting that postmenopausal women aren't getting enough vitamin K to maintain bone health.[45]
- The same study found increased excretion of

calcium in the urine in nearly 25 percent of postmenopausal women. But giving vitamin K slowed the excretion of calcium by 33 percent, which researchers suggested was an indication that bone loss had either slowed or stopped.[46]

Caution: If you're taking a blood thinner (an anticoagulant like Coumadin or warfarin), vitamin K can counteract its effects. Consult your physician before increasing your intake of vitamin K, even through dietary sources. Vitamin K can also build up in the body and cause anemia, the breakdown of red blood cells, sweats, and flushes. Taking more than 500 mcg of synthetic vitamin K is not recommended. Taking broad-spectrum antibiotics can wipe out the intestinal bacteria that produce vitamin K and put you at a high risk of deficiency. High doses of vitamin E can also interfere with vitamin K absorption.

Recommendation: Eat more dark green, leafy vegetables. You may also wish to take a 100 mcg vitamin K supplement (with a meal) once a day. Your typical vitamin-mineral supplement won't contain this much vitamin K, although some calcium supplements might. Check the labels.

Exercise

Although aerobic exercise and stretching are vital parts of any exercise program, the *only* kind of exercise that will increase or maintain your bone density is the weight-bearing kind. That's because bones respond to exercise-induced physical stress the same way muscles do—by growing bigger and stronger. Weight-bearing exercise means walking, running, jumping rope, playing sports, lifting weights, or otherwise using your bones to work against the force of gravity. Until recently, swimming was not on the list of bone-building exercises, since it's not weight bearing. But a 1987 study of 37 older female swimmers showed a mild increase in spinal density in swimmers when compared to nonathletes.[47] So while swimming may not be the best bone-building exercise, it can still provide some benefit.

An analysis of the Nurses' Health Study of 61,200 postmenopausal women, published in the *Journal of the American Medical Association* in 2002, found that postmenopausal women who walked 4 or more hours a week had a 41 percent decrease in risk of hip fracture, compared to those who exercised little or not at all. And those who exercised 8 or more hours a week enjoyed hip fracture reductions that *equaled those of women who took HRT.*[48]

Caution: As with all exercises, start slowly and increase intensity gradually. Weight-bearing exercise shouldn't hurt. If it does, you're probably doing it wrong. Get help from an expert and always listen to your body.

Recommendation: Most experts recommend engaging in weight-bearing activities for at least 20 minutes, 3–5 times a week, to promote bone health.

Lifestyle Changes

Stop Smoking
Smokers tend to have lesser bone densities and more fractures of the forearm, hip, and spine than nonsmokers.[49] This is probably due to the fact that cigarette smoking interferes with the absorption of calcium,[50] causes early menopause, and decreases

estrogen levels, all of which increase the risk of developing osteoporosis. So quit now, or risk the health and integrity of your bones.

Avoid or Limit Alcohol

Drinking excessive amounts of alcohol has been shown to promote osteoporosis, most likely because it interferes with the absorption of calcium. A study of 96 male chronic alcoholics who ranged in age from 24 to 62 found that almost half of them had osteoporosis, as did almost one-third of those under age 40![51] And these were *men*, typically a low-risk group. The effect of moderate alcohol intake is still unknown.

Recommendation: If you drink, limit it to one drink per day. If you don't drink, don't start.

Get Regular Bone Density Tests

Bone density tests can help predict your risk of developing osteoporosis and track the progress of your bones through the years. Currently, most experts recommend a low-dose radiation technique called Dual Energy X-ray Absorptiometry (DEXA), which measures the calcium content of certain bones, usually the hip and the spine. Measuring the calcium content of your spine is important because it's composed of a highly metabolic form of bone that rapidly reflects bone changes, offering a pretty good assessment of what's going on in your bones *right now*. The hip measurement is taken because it can predict your risk of hip fracture fairly accurately. *Heel ultrasound* is a less expensive kind of bone density test that some experts think rivals the DEXA for accuracy, although DEXA is still generally considered the gold standard.

Recommendation: The National Osteoporosis Foundation recommends that you get a bone density test if you fall into any of these categories:

- You're age 65 or older.
- You're postmenopausal, and have had a fracture.
- You have a parent or a sibling who fractured a wrist, hip, or vertebra.
- You weigh less than 127 pounds.
- You smoke.

Keeping an eye on the state of your bones is extremely important so that you'll know if and when you need to start taking bone-preserving medication. For some women, natural methods by themselves won't be enough to ward off osteoporosis.

Rising Stars?

- *Natural progesterone*—While estrogen helps decrease bone breakdown, it does nothing to increase bone formation, but progesterone does.[52] A deficiency in progesterone appears to play a part in bone loss. A study of 66 premenopausal women found that those with lower blood levels of progesterone had higher rates of bone loss.[53] And those with shorter luteal phases (the part of the menstrual cycle during which progesterone is produced) also lost bone more rapidly.

  The most exciting trial involving progesterone and osteoporosis was done by John R. Lee, M.D., who performed a 3-year study on 100 postmenopausal women age 38–83. Most of these women had already suffered spontaneous vertebral fractures due to osteoporosis. Each month, they applied a 3 percent progesterone cream for 12 consecutive nights, or, if they were also using estrogen, during the last 2 weeks of the estrogen regimen. During the 3-year period, none of the women in Dr. Lee's study who were given bone density tests lost *any* bone mass. (The average osteoporosis patient could be expected to lose about 4.5 percent of her bone mass during a similar period.) Even more exciting, every single woman had an *increase* in bone mass, with an overall average increase of 15.4 percent during the 3 years! And there was not one osteoporotic fracture during the entire time the women received progesterone.[54]

- *Manganese*—Manganese produces compounds called mucopolysaccharides that provide a platform for bone calcification. If there's too little manganese, the foundation of the bones will be weak and calcification won't occur properly, negatively affecting bone formation, remodeling, and repair. Women with osteoporosis often have very low blood levels of manganese.[55] A study of 14 osteoporotic women in Belgium found that their serum manganese levels were 75 percent lower than a control group of women the same age who didn't have osteoporosis.[56] The differing manganese levels were the only statistically significant difference between the two. Although there is no established daily requirement of manganese, some experts recommend a daily intake of 15–20 mg.

- *Boron*—A trace mineral found in most fruits and vegetables (particularly apples and dried fruits), boron conserves calcium and improves its utilization, helps convert vitamin D to its active form, and enhances the synthesis of estrogen and testosterone.[57] In one study, 12 postmenopausal women ages 48–82 consumed a low-boron diet for 119 days, after which they received a daily 3 mg boron supplement. The boron reduced excretion of urinary calcium by 44 percent, as well as excretion of magnesium. It also significantly increased blood levels of both testosterone and estrogen (estradiol), with blood levels of estradiol equaling those found in women taking estrogen replacement therapy![58]

Chapter Seven

Is It Hot in Here, or Is It Just Me?

Do you remember watching your mother or another older woman furiously fanning herself with a newspaper or anything else at hand, even in perfectly comfortable weather? Or did you have an aunt who had one of those little battery-operated fans that she flipped on and aimed at her face, explaining in hushed tones, "You'll understand when you get to be my age. . . ."

Now that you're near her age, you may be shocked to discover that hot flashes are becoming *your* problem. Without warning, a wave of heat can start in your chest or neck and spread upward over your face. Called hot flushes by the British, these sensations of heat can ratchet up your skin temperature as much as 8 degrees, significantly increase your heart and breathing rates, and produce drenching sweats that flow like waterworks, followed by a clammy feeling. Their nocturnal version, night sweats, can wake you from a sound sleep in the middle of the night to find yourself lying in a puddle of perspiration, with your nightclothes, sheets, and body soaked.

Hot flashes affect around 85 percent of American women,[1] most of whom will have them for more than a year.[2] They typically come and go in about 30 minutes, hitting a peak in temperature and discomfort that lasts from 30 seconds to 5 minutes. On average, hot flashes recur every 2 to 4 hours, although this varies considerably from woman to woman. These mini–heat waves usually begin during the perimenopausal years when estrogen levels begin to decline, and continue until 6 months to 5 years past menopause. But 25–50 percent of us will have them for more than 5 years,[3] and some unlucky women actually experience hot flashes for up to 15 years.

The Problem

Hot flashes are disturbing feelings of heat that seem to arise out of nowhere. They may produce nothing more than a mild to moderate feeling of warmth in the face and upper body, or they may start in the upper chest and move upward to the face and down the shoulders. Hot flashes can also trigger chills, sweating, anxiety, nausea, and dizziness, as well as heart palpitations and tingling in the fingers. Some women have hot flashes only during the day, while others get them predomiantly at night, causing drenching sweats that disturb sleep.

What Causes Hot Flashes?

No one really knows what causes hot flashes, which fall into the category of *vasomotor changes*. "Vasomotor" refers to the nerves and muscles that determine the width of the blood vessels. During a hot flash, the blood vessels dilate more than usual, bringing blood to the surface of the skin, which allows heat to escape. We do know that vasomotor changes are related to the loss of estrogen, and that giving estrogen can often eliminate the problem entirely. Two of the common theories of the origin of hot flashes:

- *A "confused" hypothalamus*—The hypothalamus is the part of the brain that controls body temperature and the sex hormones, among other things. When the hypothalamus senses that the body temperature has risen too high, it sends out signals to dilate the blood vessels directly under the skin's surface so the heat from the blood can escape. This helps to cool the body. But when the levels of estrogen and luteinizing hormone (LH) begin to drop during the years preceding menopause, the hypothalamus gets confused and starts sending out the cool down signal even when the body isn't overheated. Thus, you can be feeling perfectly fine when suddenly your skin reddens and you feel a wave of heat spreading upward across your face.

  Although you might mistake a hot flash for a fever, the rise in temperature is just skin-deep. Inside, your core body temperature may actually be falling, thanks to the escape of heat through your skin. So a hot flash is actually a simultaneous heating and cooling of the body— your skin heats up, but your inner temperature drops. In fact, some women have chills immediately after the hot flash, and others have chills plus profuse perspiration ("cold sweats").

- *LH knocking at the door*—Another theory of the

origin of hot flashes involves the hypothalamus's response to a drop in estrogen. During a regular menstrual cycle, LH prompts the release of the ripened egg from its follicle, but with the estrogen levels down, the ovaries no longer respond. So the hypothalamus begins "pounding on the door," trying to get a response from the ovaries by stimulating the release of more and more LH. In the process, the hyperactive hypothalamus wakes up a nearby area in the brain that controls body temperature, unwittingly sending it into action. The result is blasts of heat to the upper body to match the blasts of LH that are hounding the ovaries.

Hot flashes are probably a combination of both of these, plus other factors.

Who's Most Likely to Get Hot Flashes?

It's impossible to predict who will suffer from hot flashes, or whose episodes will be more severe or last longer. But some experts suggest that you will be more likely to have a problem with hot flashes if:

- *You've had surgical menopause*—Removal of the ovaries, in particular, causes an abrupt decline in hormone levels that can bring on severe hot flashes. Removal of the uterus has similar but lesser effects.
- *You're sedentary*—Women who don't exercise have three times the risk of experiencing hot flashes.[4]
- *You don't perspire easily*—Perspiration is the body's main cooling mechanism, so if it's not

working efficiently, your body will send more blood to the skin to cool itself off.

- *You're under a great deal of stress*—Increased stress levels translate to more hot flashes.[5]
- *You smoke cigarettes*—Cigarette smoking causes a drop in estrogen levels and premature menopause.[6]
- *Your mother suffered from hot flashes.*[7]

Experts are divided on the effect of body fat. Some say that thin women are more likely to have hot flashes because they have less fat in which to store estrogen, so the drop-off in estrogen production will hit them harder.[8] But others say that heavy women will have more hot flashes because fat is insulation, making it harder to release excess heat.[9]

Then there are other causes of hot flashes and night sweats that have nothing to do with menopause:

- taking selective serotonin reuptake inhibitor drugs (SSRIs), such as Prozac and Zoloft, or other medications used to treat depression
- drinking alcohol shortly before going to bed
- tuberculosis
- Hodgkin's disease

Although your hot flashes and night sweats are far and away more likely to be caused by menopausal changes, it's always a good idea to get checked out by a physician to make sure that nothing else might be causing them.

In General, You Want To:

- keep your body cool
- keep your environment cool

- keep your skin dry by wearing absorbent clothing
- avoid stressful situations

What You Can Do About It

While these suggestions won't relieve or cure the underlying problem, they can help you live with your hot flashes:

- avoid excessive heat
- avoid excess exposure to the sun, so you won't get sunburned
- avoid tight-fitting clothing that holds in the heat
- wear "cool" clothing made of cotton or other natural fibers that absorb perspiration. Avoid polyester and other synthetic materials
- dress in layers so that you can quickly shed articles of clothing when things heat up, then put them back on if you become chilled
- make sure your nightclothes and bedding are 100 percent cotton; it's absorbent and it breathes
- keep ice cubes, cold drinks, or cold foods like ice cream nearby whenever possible; sucking ice chips can cool your face in the middle of an episode
- try taking a cool shower or standing in front of an open refrigerator when a hot flash strikes
- set the thermostat in your home a little lower than usual to keep the place cool, and use the air conditioner when you're in your car

Diet

As with most conditions, what you eat can make a difference in both the frequency and severity of your hot flashes. Consider the following:

Eat Six Small Meals a Day

Try eating several small meals each day instead of three big ones, since large meals can trigger hot flashes.[10]

Watch for Trigger Foods

Foods that may spark a hot flash may include spicy ones like garlic, ginger, onions, and ground red pepper; acidic foods like tomatoes and citrus fruits; alcohol; caffeine; and sugar. Pay attention to your body's reaction to these or any other foods, and avoid them if they seem to set you off.

Drink Plenty of Water

Your body's thermostat is regulated in part by your water intake. Make sure you get those eight glasses of water every day.

Avoid Alcohol

Alcohol causes blood vessel dilation, which is likely to make your hot flashes worse. One study of alcohol's effect on hot flashes found that women who drank at least one alcoholic beverage a week were about 13 percent more likely to have hot flashes than women who didn't drink at all.[11]

Foods and Phytochemicals

Black Cohosh (Cimicifuga racemosa)

An herb belonging to the buttercup family, black cohosh is one of the oldest herbal remedies for "female troubles," used by Native Americans to treat menstrual discomfort and the pains of childbirth. Since the 1700s, black cohosh has been used in Western civilizations to treat the symptoms of menopause.

This herb is the active ingredient in Remifemin, the most widely used and extensively studied natural treatment for menopause in existence.[12] Most of the double-blind, placebo-controlled studies of black cohosh were conducted in Germany, where it's been found to be as effective as estrogen in relieving hot flashes, and is officially approved as a viable treatment for menopausal symptoms, PMS, and menstrual disorders.

It's unclear exactly how black cohosh works to relieve hot flashes and other menopausal symptoms, but some evidence suggests that it suppresses the action of luteinizing hormone (LH).[13] Animal studies[14] and test tube studies[15] indicate that it does not appear to act as a phytoestrogen, which means it probably won't exacerbate estrogen-dependent cancers like breast cancer. Some of the scientific evidence of the effectiveness of black cohosh includes the following:

- An early study with black cohosh was performed by more than 100 physicians working with more than 600 women. After 8 weeks of use, an extract of black cohosh had produced obvious improvement in more than 80 percent of the women, including a reduction in hot flashes and perspiration.[16]
- A German study involving 60 women with hot flashes following hysterectomy divided the women into four groups. One group took black cohosh, the second took a form of estrogen called estriol, the third took conjugated estrogens, and the fourth took estrogen plus a progestin. Black cohosh reduced the number and intensity of hot flashes just as effectively as any of the three forms of estrogen.[17]

- In one double-blind, randomized, placebo-controlled study, black cohosh was compared to placebo for 12 weeks in menopausal women between 46 and 58 years of age suffering from vasomotor changes and psychological complaints. Hot flashes and psychological symptoms both decreased significantly, down to levels seen in patients not suffering from menopausal complaints.[18]
- A review study that looked at eight human studies involving an extract of black cohosh concluded that it is safe and effective for treating menopausal symptoms.[19]

Cautions: Although many studies of black cohosh have found it safe and effective, none have lasted longer than 6 months; thus, we don't know if it's safe to use for longer time periods. Potential adverse reactions include gastrointestinal disturbances, headache, and weight gain. An overdose may trigger perspiration, nausea, vomiting, dizziness, and other problems.

Recommendations: A typical dose of black cohosh is 20–40 mg of a standardized extract. There's no need to take more than 40 mg. One study found that daily doses of either 40 mg or 127 mg were equally effective.[20]

Soy or Soybeans

Did you know that the Japanese have no word for "hot flashes"? That's because only about 25 percent of Japanese women ever experience this phenomenon,[21] compared to up to 85 percent of North American women. Many researchers believe that this is because of the high intake of soy and soy isoflavones in Japan—125–150 mg of soy isoflavones per day, as opposed to the average American intake of about 1 mg.

Soy isoflavones are phytoestrogens that act like a mild dose of estrogen in the body. One study comparing the urinary isoflavone content of a group of women found that those who ate soy excreted 100 to 1,000 times more isoflavonoids than nonsoy eaters—enough to have a biological effect on those with low estrogen levels.[22] In fact, just one cup of soybeans (300 mg of isoflavones) provides the equivalent of about 0.45 mg of conjugated estrogens or one tablet of Premarin.[23]

In 2000, the American College of Obstetricians and Gynecologists gave their official stamp of approval to soy for relief of vasomotor symptoms, stating that "Soy and isoflavones may be helpful in the short term (2 years or less) for menopausal symptoms such as hot flashes and night sweats."[24] This comes after repeated studies showing that soy really does help ease these symptoms:

- A double-blind study tested the effects of soy and wheat on hot flashes. Fifty-eight postmenopausal women who had at least fourteen hot flashes a week were given dietary supplementation with either soy flour or wheat flour. Twelve weeks later, *both* groups showed significant reductions in hot flashes and overall menopausal symptom scores. But while wheat flour reduced the number of hot flashes by 25 percent, soy flour reduced them by 40 percent.[25]
- From *Menopause* comes a study of 75 women, ages 43–53, who took either a soy isoflavone extract or a placebo. After 16 weeks, those taking the soy enjoyed a 61 percent reduction in hot

flashes, compared to only a 21 percent reduction among those taking the placebo.[26]

- Japanese researchers looked specifically at fermented soy products such as tempeh and miso in their 1999 study of soy and hot flashes. Two hundred and eighty-four women, ranging in age from 40 to 59, completed a health and diet questionnaire. Analysis of their answers showed a "reverse relationship" between consumption of fermented soy products and the severity of hot flashes. That is, the greater the amount of fermented soy products ingested, the less severe the hot flashes.[27]

(See "Isoflavones in Foods," page 117, in the section on "Soy and Soybeans" in Chapter 6.)

Caution: See Caution, page 59, in "Soy or Soybeans" section in Chapter 4.

Recommendation: To reduce hot flashes, consume up to 150 mg of isoflavones *in food form* every day. Do not exceed 150 mg, the upper limit found in the Japanese diet, and avoid taking isoflavone supplements as their safety has not been confirmed.

Exercise

It's not clear whether physical activity itself helps ease hot flashes, or if it's just staying in shape that does the trick. We do know, however, that those who engage in regular, moderate, and reasonable physical activity are generally healthier than their sedentary counterparts, and that may play a big part in their lack of hot flashes:

- Swedish researchers looked into the link between physical activity and vasomotor symptoms, including hot flashes. Their survey of 793 women with natural (nonsurgical) menopause revealed that only 5 percent of women who were very physically active had severe hot flashes, compared to three times that number in the relatively inactive group.[28]

- Another Swedish study found that more exercise was related to fewer and less intense hot flashes. In fact, the physically active women in the study had about half as many moderate-to-severe hot flashes as the control group. And most of those who exercised approximately 3.5 hours a week had no hot flashes at all.[29]

- A study involving both premenopausal and postmenopausal women found that both had higher estrogen levels after participating in an aerobic training program, and more than half of the postmenopausal women enjoyed a decrease in hot flash intensity.[30]

Recommendation: Exercise regularly. Even if it doesn't directly help reduce the number or severity of your hot flashes, it may help by improving your self-image and feeling of control. And both of these can give you a more positive attitude toward menopause, which could help reduce the severity of your symptoms.

Lifestyle Changes

Stop Smoking

If you're already feeling too hot, does it make sense to light up? A study published in the *Journal of Women's Health* examined the link between hot flashes and various demographic and behavioral factors, arriving at the conclusion that hot flashes are definitely linked to cigarette smoking.[31]

Smoking can constrict the blood vessels, which means it might make your body fight against itself during a hot flash. Remember, your hypothalamus mistakenly believes that your body is overheated, so it orders the blood vessels near the skin to open wider so that heat from the blood can dissipate through the skin. By constricting those vessels through smoking, you may prolong the hot flash by making it difficult for the blood to throw off its excess heat.

Recommendations: Stop smoking. Give up cigarettes, cigars, and pipes—now.

Lose Those Extra Pounds

No one is quite sure which is more likely to cause hot flashes: being slim or being heavy. Some say heavy women have fewer hot flashes because fatty tissue is a source of estrogen, and extra fat equals higher circulating levels of this hormone. Others say heavy women have more hot flashes because their bodies have more insulation.

But some evidence suggests that maintaining ideal body weight can help with hot flashes. For example, an Italian study of 181 women found that women with greater body weight are more likely to suffer hot flashes and sweating.[32] Others have suggested that maintaining ideal body weight can help reduce hot flash severity through an entirely different mechanism—the mind. A recent study looked at the link between self-esteem and menopausal symptoms.[33] Among the women participating, those who were pleased with their physical appearance or had higher self-esteem tended to have less trouble with menopausal symptoms. Since satisfaction with your physical appearance and higher self-esteem are often linked to maintaining a healthy weight, it would probably be a helpful strategy for hot flash control to drop those extra pounds.

Relax

While you can't do anything about the fact that you're going through "the change," you can alter your attitude toward it. Specifically, you can relax mentally and accept what's happening to you without getting too stressed. Various types of relaxation can help us shed some stress and soften our symptoms. The relaxation response, a physiological quieting that brings about lower heart and breathing rates, a relaxation of the muscles throughout the body, slower brain-wave patterns, and a reduction in stress hormone levels, can be summoned by methods like meditation, yoga, and progressive relaxation. Regularly practicing the relaxation response can bring big health benefits, including a reduction in the frequency and intensity of your hot flashes:

- Researchers from Harvard Medical School's Mind/Body Medical Institute tested the effects of the relaxation response on 33 women between the ages of 44 and 66. All of the participants were postmenopausal and in good health. This study showed that daily use of the relaxation response led to a significant drop in the intensity of hot flashes, as well as the amount of tension, anxiety and depression.[34]
- Swedish researchers conducted a small study looking at the effects of applied relaxation on postmenopausal hot flashes. Their 12-week study found that practicing applied relaxation decreased the number of hot flashes.[35]

Recommendation: You may be able to stop a hot flash in progress just by sitting in a quiet place, breathing deeply, and relaxing for several minutes. Find some time each day to practice the relaxation response. You can get there via many pathways: applied relaxation, aromatherapy, autogenic training, biofeedback, cognitive behavioral therapy, deep breathing, meditation, prayer, progressive relaxation, qi gong, relaxation tapes, self-hypnosis, soothing music, tai chi, warm baths, yoga, or whatever it takes to keep you cool.

Natural Progesterone

According to *The Merck Manual of Medical Information*, women who can't take estrogen may be given progesterone to reduce the discomfort of hot flashes.[36] Why? Hot flashes are due to a lack of hormonal response to the promptings of the hypothalamus. The hypothalamus signals the pituitary, and the pituitary starts bombarding the ovaries with blasts of LH to get them to release an egg. These blasts of hormone may be the cause of hot flashes. But when progesterone levels are raised, the pituitary will stop trying to force the ovaries to produce an egg. That's because under normal conditions progesterone levels rise markedly once an egg is produced. So the presence of progesterone fools the pituitary into thinking an egg has been released and it's time to relax—no need for hot flashes.[37]

Another reason that progesterone may help quell hot flashes is that it's a precursor to estrogen—that is, estrogen can be manufactured in the body from progesterone.

- A review of five randomized controlled trials including 257 women found that those taking synthetic progesterone had significant reductions in hot flashes compared to those taking a placebo.[38]

- But natural progesterone appears to work just as well. A randomized controlled trial of 102 women found that a daily application of 20 mg of progesterone cream to the skin improved or eliminated vasomotor symptoms in 83 percent of the treatment group, compared to 19 percent in the placebo group.[39]

Caution: Although progesterone reputedly has no side effects, more study is needed. Don't confuse natural progesterone with wild yam cream. While natural progesterone can be synthesized in a laboratory from wild yams, unless this laboratory conversion takes place, the body can't utilize the active ingredients found in wild yams.

Recommendation: A typical dose of transdermal progesterone is 20 mg (or about ¼ tsp) of a 1.6 percent cream.[40] Consult your physician before using progesterone cream to alleviate hot flashes or any other menopausal symptoms.

Rising Stars?

Below are a few other substances that may prove to be valuable, when more research is conducted on their effects on human subjects.

- *Vitamin E*—Back in the 1940s, controlled clinical trials found that vitamin E was effective in relieving hot flashes and worked by stabilizing the blood vessels so they wouldn't dilate as much in response to hormonal changes.[41] Since that time, however, the topic has been ignored, leaving us with no current studies. However, many experts recommend 800 IU of vitamin E daily to relieve hot flashes. Once the hot flashes simmer down, you may want to reduce the dose to 400 IU.

- *Dong quai*—Although we don't have solid scientific evidence that this herb can help ameliorate hot flashes, a great many women report that it has helped them.
- *Hesperidin*—One of the flavonoids found in oranges and lemons, hesperidin was tested in a placebo-controlled study. When hesperidin and vitamin C were given to more than 90 women suffering from hot flashes, symptoms were relieved in 53 percent and reduced in 34 percent.[42]
- *Red clover*—Red clover, which contains isoflavones, acts like a weak estrogen in your body. It's found in Promensil, a supplement that reduces hot flashes in some women, although the results of studies have been mixed. However, some studies[43] have found that red clover caused breast cancer cells to multiply and grow as effectively as real estrogen—so be wary.

Chapter Eight

The Emotional Roller Coaster

The menopausal years are jam-packed with stressors that can leave you anxious, irritable, depressed, or fatigued. You may be working full time; taking care of elderly, ailing parents; shepherding teenagers through turbulent years; coping with "empty nest syndrome"; wondering how you're going to pay for the kids' college tuition, weddings, or other big expenditures, or dealing with extreme changes in important relationships (including separation, divorce, and death). Or maybe you're doing all of the above. Yikes! And your changing hormone levels can make your feelings even more intense because of the numerous estrogen and progesterone receptors in the brain, where these hormones "plug in" and influence biochemistry, physiology and mood. As your estrogen and progesterone supplies wane, you'll feel the difference. Then factor in testosterone, which takes on a greater presence in relation to your dwindling female hormones, and you'll find yourself dealing with a brand-new biochemical mix that can bring on emotional changes that feel like a permanent case of PMS.

The Problem

Many peri- and postmenopausal women suffer from anxiety, depression, irritability, or other emotional changes. These can range in severity from mildly annoying to life-threatening, and may be triggered by a variety of problems, including hormonal changes and stress.

The good news is that the moodiness, depression, anxiety, and irritability experienced during the peri- and postmenopausal years rarely develop into serious psychological troubles. But that doesn't mean these feelings can't seriously affect your relationships, ability to work, self-esteem, and quality of life while they last. If you experience severe emotional upheavals or mood changes that linger for more than a week or two, see a mental health professional. Most of these problems can be successfully treated without drugs, although more serious problems may require some medication. Either way, get help before things spiral out of control.

Note: The recommendations in this chapter are designed for women who experience mild emotional changes that may respond to changes in diet and lifestyle, not for those with serious emotional problems.

How Do Hormones Cause Emotional Changes?

Although estrogen deficiency per se hasn't been proven to cause "menopausal moods," we know that fluctuations in hormone levels do alter the way you feel. This is because hormones work together in a delicate balance that can easily be thrown out of whack, particularly during the perimenopausal years when estrogen and/or progesterone levels can rise and fall several times during a single day. Anxiety, depression, irritability, and other emotional changes can result from the following hormonal states:

- *Estrogen dominance/progesterone deficiency*—During premenopause and perimenopause, when ovulation becomes sporadic or disappears entirely, progesterone production falls to practically nothing. Yet estrogen production may stay at normal or even high levels, causing an imbalance between these two hormones called *estrogen dominance*. This can continue to happen *after* menopause in heavy women, since a certain amount of estrogen will continue to be manufactured via the fat cells. Whatever the cause, there's just too much estrogen relative to progesterone in the body.

  Estrogen dominance (or progesterone deficiency) can cause anxiety, depression, emotional hypersensitivity, fatigue, low blood sugar, migraine headaches, and sleeplessness. Too much estrogen also lowers magnesium levels, which can cause sugar cravings and mood swings. And estrogen grabs and holds water, resulting in weight gain, bloating, and breast tenderness, all of which can contribute to a depressed mood.

- *Lack of estrogen*—Estrogen plays a part in instructing the brain to increase levels of *serotonin*, the brain's natural tranquilizer and antidepressant (often called the "feel-good hormone").

Without enough estrogen, serotonin levels can plummet, leaving you feeling depressed and anxious. Too little estrogen can also contribute to emotional changes by bringing on hot flashes and night sweats that disrupt your sleep. And if you're not getting enough sleep because you're waking up several times a night on fire or drenched in sweat, you have good reason to be depressed, fatigued, anxious, and irritable.

- *"Unmasking" of testosterone*—During and after menopause, not only is the absolute level of estrogen lower than it has been in decades, the relative level is also lower compared to other hormones, particularly testosterone. Up until now testosterone has flowed through your body like a little stream dwarfed by cascades of female hormones. But when the female hormones dwindle down to a mere trickle, the testosterone stream suddenly begins to look like a river in comparison, influencing the body in new ways. Suddenly, you may find yourself feeling more aggressive, angry, or irritable than before. On the positive side, you may also experience an increase in your sex drive.

- *Stress hormones*—Chronic stress interferes with normal hormone function; worsens mood swings; increases muscle tension, sugar cravings, insomnia, and pain; and leads to exhaustion. One reason is that when you're stressed, your adrenal glands release hormones that speed up your heart and breathing rate, tense your muscles, and release sugar into your bloodstream for quick energy. *Cortisol,* one of these hormones, is produced at twenty times its normal rate when you're under stress and is manufactured at the expense of your progesterone supply. So if you're dealing with chronic stress, you can use up your progesterone supply in a hurry and throw your body into a semipermanent state of estrogen dominance.

Who's Most Likely to Experience Emotional Changes?

Menopausal mood disturbances are most likely to surface in the woman who:

- experienced mood changes during PMS
- had postpartum depression
- abruptly stopped taking estrogen replacement therapy
- had a hysterectomy or oophorectomy (removal of the ovaries)
- experienced a long and troublesome perimenopause

A Brief Look at the Big Three—Anxiety, Depression, and Irritability

Anxiety, depression and irritability strike all of us from time to time, no matter where we are in the life cycle. But the average woman in her forties or fifties is particularly at risk due to her changing hormones, plus the radical changes in her relationships, family and work responsibilities, health, financial status, and appearance that can go along with this time of life. But when does reasonable worry become anxiety? Or natural sadness become depression? Or justifiable irritation become unreasonable? In other words, at what point do normal, necessary emotions become destructive? To answer these questions, let's take a closer look at each of them.

Anxiety

Anxiety can generally be described as "invented worry." It's an exaggerated fear that may begin with a genuine concern, but gets blown out of proportion. While fear is a healthy response to real or potential danger, anxiety involves excessive amounts of fear in response to dangers that may not even exist. For example, you're driving down a street, past many driveways and alleys, and you suddenly become very worried that a car may hurtle out of one of them and smash into you.

Potential signs of anxiety include:

- a generalized feeling of uneasiness
- being on the alert for danger at all times. Even casual remarks can trigger your alarm bells.
- rapid heart rate
- rapid breathing
- difficulty sleeping
- difficulty concentrating

Chronic anxiety is worry that consumes your life and serves no beneficial purpose. It can make it impossible for you to attend to your normal activities and seriously interfere with your ability to enjoy life. If you're troubled by anxiety, a mental health professional can help you identify the internal stressors that set off the attacks and teach you some coping mechanisms to make it easier to deal with them.

Depression

We've all had feelings of hopelessness and helplessness from time to time, which are normal reactions to difficult or frustrating situations. Depression that strikes during or after difficult times (e.g., after the death of a loved one or the loss of job) is called *reactive depression*, and it's to be expected. Reactive depression arises in response to a particular situation, has a certain "shelf life," and eventually resolves itself. Prayer and reflection, some sessions with a psychologist, a deep talk with a sympathetic friend, and time spent with friends or family can help ease this kind of depression and get you back on your feet again.

But sometimes the feelings of doom and gloom may be stronger than they should be, last longer than the situation warrants, and cloud your mind for no apparent reason. This is known as *endogenous depression*, the kind of depression that arises from within, rather than in response to an event. Endogenous depression is much more serious than reactive depression. Since it has no apparent cause, it's much harder to treat and a lot more likely to hang around indefinitely. But whether it's reactive or endogenous, if depression stays with you for more than two weeks and you find yourself unable to take pleasure in the things you used to enjoy, you're probably suffering from a major depressive episode that requires treatment.

Other signs of major depression include:

- crying
- difficulty sleeping
- significant changes in appetite, with a loss or gain in weight

- loss of interest in sex
- inability to laugh
- brooding
- difficulty concentrating
- severe fatigue
- feelings of sadness, worthlessness or extreme guilt
- hopelessness
- thoughts of suicide

Ongoing depression can make it all but impossible for you to handle your family responsibilities, your work, and your social life. In extreme cases, it can be life-threatening. If you suffer from depression, even if you think it's only a mild form, seek professional help. It's better to overreact and call for help too soon than to wait too long and run the risk of harming yourself.

Irritability/Chronic Anger

We all get angry from time to time, usually in response to frustration: you want to get somewhere in a hurry and someone gets in your way. But often this kind of anger recedes quickly once the situation is resolved. Chronic anger occurs when a person believes that life is nothing but one frustrating event after another. In his book *Psychological Symptoms*, Frank J. Bruno, Ph.D., says that chronic anger has three main attributes:[1]

- *It's pathological*—It poisons the person's life and possibly brings on physical illness.
- *It's excessive*—It's an overboard reaction to a frustrating incident.

- *It's irrational*—It involves an idea that's neither logical nor reasonable.

If you're constantly hurrying; impatient; unable to relax, play, or enjoy vacations; or if you're verbally aggressive; you often think of others as stupid; lazy, or incompetent; or if you speak to others in an abrupt, harsh manner, you may be chronically angry. It's possible that you're using anger to mask anxiety. Or you may be easily aroused physiologically, or you've found that getting angry and bullying others is an easy way to get what you want. A mental health professional can help you discover the unconscious motivations behind your anger, find ways to avoid frustrating situations, and improve your communication skills.

In General, You Want To:

- "smooth out" moods that seem to be out of proportion to their precipitating events
- avoid letting a "bad mood" become a chronic emotional problem by getting help from a mental health professional if moods last more than two weeks

What You Can Do About It

Assuming your emotional changes are mild, temporary, and non–life threatening, there are several things you can do to help "smooth down" your moods.

Diet

In general, consuming a nutritious, balanced diet and eating several times a day can help lessen mood swings. Then pay particular attention to these diet tips:

Eat Plenty of Complex Carbohydrates

Complex carbohydrates, found in whole grains, fruits, and vegetables, aid in the uptake of the amino acid tryptophan into the brain. There, the tryptophan is converted into serotonin, the hormone that promotes a feeling of well-being and can relieve depression, irritability, and insomnia. This process takes place rapidly after you eat carbohydrates, so just having a piece of bread or a few crackers could help elevate your mood within a couple of minutes. Although simple carbohydrates (sugar, fructose, etc.) will have the same effect, the quick rise and fall of blood sugar can leave you more irritable and depressed than when you started. Stick with complex carbohydrates for longer-lasting mood elevation.

Maintain Consistent Levels of Blood Glucose

Your brain is fueled almost entirely by glucose, so it's not surprising that low blood sugar levels would have a major impact on your moods. Irritability, weakness, headaches, fainting, depression, and illogical fears are all signs of too little glucose in the brain.[2] You can bring on low blood sugar by dieting, fasting, or otherwise eating too infrequently, or by eating too many sugary treats (especially if you eat them as snacks with no accompanying high-protein, high-fiber foods). Your body has to do less work to break down sugar (a simple carbohydrate) than it does to break down complex carbohydrates. This means that the glucose from a candy bar, for example, will be released into your bloodstream almost immediately after you eat it. In response, your blood sugar will skyrocket, which prompts your body to release a surge of insulin to "clean up" all that sugar. Unfortunately, the insulin often does its job too well, and your blood sugar levels end up plunging lower than ever, taking your good mood along with it.

To maintain steady glucose levels, try the following:

- avoid eating sugar or foods containing large amounts of sugar (candy, cakes, pies, jelly, honey, fructose, corn syrup, etc.)
- eat 5–6 small meals a day, so that glucose will be gradually and steadily released into your bloodstream throughout the day
- distribute your carbohydrate intake throughout the day
- to slow the absorption of glucose, eat foods containing protein, fat, or fiber when eating a high sugar food. Fruit should not be eaten by itself— add some cottage cheese or a spoonful of peanut butter.

Watch Your Caffeine Intake

Caffeine revs you up—that's its main attraction. But it can also make you irritable, jittery, and prone to low blood sugar. Caffeine stimulates a release of insulin from the pancreas that can gobble up too much blood sugar, leaving you hungry, craving sweets, on edge, and light-headed. Limit your intake of caffeine-containing beverages to one or two per day. (See the "Take Care with Caffeine" section in Chapter 5, page 86.)

Avoid or Limit Alcohol

Alcohol is a central nervous system depressant, so those who have problems with depression should avoid it completely. It lessens inhibitions, increasing a tendency toward irritability or displays of anger in some people. This can be compounded by the fact that alcohol is derived from sugar, leading to blood sugar rises and falls that increase irritability, anxiety, and poor moods. It takes substantial amounts of B vitamins, vitamin C, magnesium, calcium, potassium, and zinc to convert alcohol into energy, so the more you drink, the more likely you are to deplete your supply of these important vitamins and minerals.

Foods, Phytochemicals, and Amino Acids

DL-Phenylalanine (DLPA)

Back in the 1970s, researchers at Johns Hopkins University were surprised to discover that there were morphine receptors in the brain: that is, that the brain was designed to interact with morphine. This was an odd finding, since morphine isn't a naturally occurring substance in the body. The only logical answer was that there was a type of morphine inside the body that used those morphine receptors. That "morphine" within the body turned out to be the *endorphins*, natural substances that help to block chronic pain and modulate mood.

Further research established that the body continually builds and destroys these endorphin molecules, and that taking the amino acid phenylalanine could protect the endorphins from routine destruction, allowing their levels to build and elevate depressed moods. For example:

- Fifteen patients suffering from depression were given phenylalanine twice daily. Within five days, the depressive symptoms were substantially reduced in 10 of the 15. And for those 5 who were not helped by phenylalanine, the supplement worked later on with their standard medications, making them more effective.[3]
- European researchers studied 23 people suffering from endogenous depression, the kind that seems to come from nowhere and refuses to leave. These people had not been helped by the medications they had taken previously. Two weeks after being given phenylalanine, 17 of the 23 had returned to a normal emotional state.[4]
- In a larger study, 370 people suffering from endogenous depression were treated with a form of phenylalanine called DLPA. Within 15 days, 73 percent had returned to a "normal affective state." Within 2 months, 80 percent enjoyed a normal affective state, and 15 percent showed improvement.[5]

Cautions:

- Those with phenylketonuria (PKU) or alkaptonuria should not take phenylalanine, as they cannot metabolize the amino acid normally. Neither should anyone on a phenylalanine-restricted diet take phenylalanine.
- Taking phenylalanine along with monoamine oxidase inhibitors (MAOIs), selegiline (Eldepryl), levodopa, or neuroleptic drugs may be dangerous.
- Those with hypertension, schizophrenia, stroke, or tyrosinemia or tyrosinuria should only use phenylalanine under a physician's supervision.

- DLPA is not quick acting, like an aspirin. Several weeks may pass before you feel its effects.

Recommendations: The form of phenylalanine that appears to work best for depression is called DLPA (DL-phenylalanine). While there is no established dose, typical doses are 150–200 mg DLPA per day.

5-hydroxytryptophan (5-HTP)

Depression has been linked to low levels of serotonin,[6] which is manufactured in the body through a combination of the amino acid tryptophan, carbohydrates, vitamin B_6, and magnesium. The current FDA-approved form of this amino acid supplement is 5-hydroxytryptophan (5-HTP). Taking 5-HTP increases tryptophan levels in the brain and may increase brain serotonin levels. Low levels of brain serotonin have been linked to aggressive behavior[7] and depression, so pumping up your brain's supply of this "feel-good hormone" may make you feel calmer and less depressed.

The results of studies testing whether 5-HTP boosts serotonin levels in the brain and hence relieves depression have been encouraging:

- An early European double-blind study published in 1977 compared 5-HTP to the antidepressant imipramine. The researchers found that 5-HTP performed as effectively as the drug in relieving depression.[8]
- Swiss scientists enrolled 25 patients in a study looking at the depression-relieving effects of 5-HTP when taken alone or combined with another substance. They concluded that 5-HTP was just as helpful in relieving depression as traditional antidepressants.[9]

- The Cochrane Database, which produces highly respected reviews of the medical literature, published a review of studies of 5-hydroxytryptophan and its sister substance, tryptophan, in 2002. The reviewers concluded that while there were only a small number of studies available for review, 5-HTP and tryptophan were both effective for relieving depression.[10]

Note: 5-hydroxytryptophan is related to tryptophan, but isn't the same thing. In the late 1980s, a batch of tainted tryptophan supplements imported from Japan caused serious side effects, including the death of several people. Although tryptophan supplements per se have never been proven dangerous (in this case it was simply a tainted batch), this form of the amino acid has since been banned in the United States. 5-hydroxytryptophan is FDA approved.

Caution: Taking large amounts of 5-HTP may cause anorexia, nausea, vomiting, and diarrhea. 5-HTP should be used cautiously with medications such as carbidopa and serotonin agonists. There have been a few reports associating 5-HTP with blood disorders.

Recommendations: There is no established dose for 5-HTP. For depression, typical doses range from 100 to 300 mg per day.

Kava (Piper methysticum)

Captain Cook was the first Westerner to take note of kava, which is used as a ceremonial tranquilizing beverage in many areas of the South Pacific. As an herb, kava is used to alleviate anxiety, insomnia, restlessness and the effects of stress. It has been approved as a remedy for anxiety, agitation and tension by the German Commission E, the German equivalent of the U.S. Food and Drug Administration.

Kava's active ingredients include the *kavalactones*, which, among other things, relax skeletal muscles. Research into the herb's ability to calm anxiety has yielded encouraging results:

- Researchers gave 101 people suffering from anxiety disorders either a kava extract or a placebo for approximately 6 months. By the eighth week, the volunteers taking the kava extract showed a lessening in anxiety and continued to improve through the course of the study.[11] It's interesting to note that the patients in this study did not develop a tolerance to kava, as often happens with standard anxiety medications.
- A double-blind study tested the efficacy of a kava extract in 58 patients with various anxiety and neurotic disorders. After the first week, those taking the kava enjoyed a significant decline in anxiety compared to those taking the placebo, and the advantage of kava over placebo grew as the study continued.[12]
- Back in 1990, a proprietary brand of kava was compared to oxazepam, a standard medication for anxiety, in 38 patients suffering from anxiety. The researchers concluded that the herb was just as effective as the drug.[13]
- In sum, these studies suggest that kava is an effective, short-term treatment for anxiety.[14]

Caution: Kava's potential side effects include drowsiness, mild gastrointestinal problems, headaches, dizziness, equilibrium disturbances, and, in rare cases, allergic reactions involving the skin. Kava can cause drowsiness and interfere with the ability to drive or operate machinery. Long-term use of large doses of kava (up to 100 times the standard therapeutic dose) can lead to "kava dermopathy" or dermatitis, possibly accompanied by eye irritation. Using kava in conjunction with alcohol, drugs that suppress the central nervous system, or other herbs that have sedative properties will increase the risk of side effects.

Recommendations: The German Commission E has approved daily use of 60–120 mg of kavalactones, the principal psychoactive compounds in kava, for up to 3 months.

Omega-3 Fatty Acids

My father always used to say, "Eat your fish. It's brain food." And he may have been right. A large percentage of your brain is made up of fats (brain lipids), and your diet is reflected in your brain lipid content. This is shown in laboratory tests with rats, who show a difference in the contents of their brain lipids after only a few weeks on experimental diets.[15]

Eating omega-3 fatty acids, the kind of fat found in cold water fish and flax oil, may be able to help stabilize moods. In one study of patients with bipolar disorder (manic/depression), taking 9.6 grams of omega-3 fatty acids in supplement form each day helped stabilize their conditions.[16] And students under stress taking final examinations who took omega-3 supplements showed decreased levels of aggression.[17]

Cautions: See Cautions in the Omega-3 Fatty Acids/Fish section, page 53, in Chapter 4.

Recommendation: Although there is no set dosage for stabilizing moods with omega-3 fatty acids, 1–3 grams per day is reasonable.

St.-John's-Wort (Hypericum perforatum)

Although the ancient Greeks used St.-John's-wort to treat demonic possession, extracts of the herb are currently used to fight depression. In Germany, St.-John's-wort is the most commonly prescribed antidepressant in the country. Numerous studies have tested the herb's effectiveness against depression:

- A study conducted by German researchers compared an extract of St.-John's-wort to a standard antidepressant drug called imipramine in 324 mild to moderately depressed patients. They found that the St.-John's-wort extract was just as strong as imipramine, but was better tolerated.[18]
- A similar study, appearing in the *British Medical Journal* in 1999, compared St.-John's-wort extract to imipramine and to a placebo in 263 moderately depressed patients. St.-John's-wort extract was found to be at least as effective as the drug, and more effective than a placebo.[19]
- Researchers used statistical methods to combine the results of 23 different randomized experimental trials, and concluded that St.-John's-wort is stronger than a placebo for treatment of mild to moderate depression.[20]

Extracts of St.-John's-wort have been safely used in clinical studies lasting up to 2 months. And although St.-John's-wort has been used extensively in Germany, there have been no reports of serious toxicity problems.

Caution: Potential side effects include insomnia, restlessness, irritability, fatigue, and headache. In theory, mixing St.-John's-wort with other herbs with sedative properties can increase both the strength and the side effects of the herbs. St.-John's-wort may interact with antidepressants, narcotics, oral contraceptives, warfarin, and other drugs. Major depression, bipolar disorder, and infertility may be worsened by the use of St.-John's-wort.

Recommendation: There is no set dose of St.-John's-wort for relief of depression. In many studies, researchers used an extract standardized at 0.3 percent hypericin, with doses of 300 mg three times a day.

SAMe

SAMe (S-adenosyl-L-methionine) is a naturally occurring compound in the body that comes from the amino acid methionine. It aids in the manufacture of hormones, neurotransmitters, and proteins and guards against DNA mutation. When given in pharmacological doses (up to 1 gram per day), SAMe can also combat depression.[21] It does this, in part, by increasing serotonin production.[22]

- Italian researchers conducted two studies looking at the effects of SAMe on major depressive episodes. In one study patients were given either an injection of SAMe or the drug imipramine; in the other, patients received either an oral dose of SAMe or imipramine. In both studies, SAMe proved to be as effective in relieving depression as the drug, but caused fewer side effects.[23]
- A 2002 study compared injections of SAMe to imipramine in 293 patients with major depression. Half were given SAMe for four weeks, the other half the antidepressant medicine. Again, SAMe worked as well as the drug, but was much better tolerated.[24]
- Fifteen patients suffering from depression were randomly assigned to receive either 800 mg of

SAMe twice a day or a placebo. Three weeks later, two-thirds of those taking the SAMe reported a 50 percent improvement on their Hamilton Depression scale scores, compared to only 17 percent of those taking the placebo.[25]

Cautions: SAMe may cause headaches or nausea and other gastrointestinal side effects, particularly at higher doses. SAMe can also trigger anxiety, mania, and hypomania. It should not be used in conjunction with antidepressants.

Recommendation: There is no set dosage for SAMe. Some studies suggest that doses of 200–1,600 mg per day may be effective for relieving depression, although some may need higher doses.[26]

Vitamins and Minerals

B Vitamins

We've long known that the B vitamins are connected to moods. Many people suffering from major depression and other psychiatric disorders have low blood levels of B vitamins, and in alcoholics, depression is a classic symptom of alcohol-induced deficiencies of thiamin, niacin, B_6, and folic acid. Way back in 1957, nine healthy young men were deliberately given a diet deficient in thiamin (formerly known as vitamin B_1), and five of them became markedly depressed and irritable.[27] Conversely, in four double-blind studies, improvement in thiamin status was found to improve mood.[28]

Vitamin B_6 is particularly important to mood because of its role in nervous system function and synthesis of the mood-elevating hormone serotonin. Deficiencies in B_6 result in depression, anxiety, irritability, and insomnia. Supplementation of this vitamin has been found to be helpful in treating PMS-related depression,[29] which may originate from low levels of serotonin. It makes sense to get plenty of B_6 in your diet by eating such foods as meat, fish, poultry, bananas, cantaloupe, broccoli, and spinach.

Depression has also been associated with deficiencies in both vitamin B_{12} and folic acid.[30] Deficiencies in folic acid can cause a decline in levels of the brain's natural antidepressant SAMe, which brings about clinical depression in some people.[31] Giving folic acid supplements to depressed patients who are deficient in this vitamin (which may be as many as 30 percent of psychiatric patients)[32] can help them recover faster.[33]

Caution: The B vitamins work together as a group. Don't overload on any single vitamin or you will upset the balance.

Recommendation: To make sure that you're getting adequate amounts of the B vitamins, eat a balanced diet that includes foods rich in these nutrients, including beans, spinach, broccoli, cauliflower, avocado, orange juice, bananas, chicken breast, brown rice, wheat germ, peanuts, dried sunflower seeds, and fish. A balanced B-vitamin supplement will supply 50–100 mg each of thiamin, riboflavin, and B_6 and will also contain niacin, pantothenic acid, folic acid, and B_{12}.

Calcium

Calcium, a mineral essential to nerve function and cellular metabolism, may also play a part in regulating mood. In one 4-week study, giving depressed patients 1,000 mg of calcium gluconate plus 600 IU of vitamin D twice a day resulted in significant mood elevation compared to a placebo.[34] A deficiency in calcium, on the other hand, can result in symptoms such as anxiety, fatigue, tension, insomnia, and neurosis.

Estrogen regulates calcium metabolism, and alterations in calcium status have long been associated with mood disorders, including depression and anxiety. A review of clinical trials of calcium supplementation and PMS found that taking calcium can alleviate mood disturbances.[35] Another study found that increasing calcium intake reduced poor mood, concentration, and behavior symptoms in women with normal menstrual cycles, no matter what time of the month.[36] Although these studies don't pertain directly to menopause, they do indicate a calcium-induced effect on mood. And since you are probably taking in plenty of calcium already (in food or supplement form), mood regulation is just another reason to keep it up.

Cautions: See cautions in calcium section in Chapter 6, page 119.

Recommendation: See recommendation for calcium intake in Chapter 6, page 119.

Exercise

Regular exercise (especially aerobic exercise) helps ease stress, relax the muscles, decrease insomnia, and increase the production of endorphins, the body's natural mood elevators. And according to many studies, exercise also has a profound effect on one's overall outlook.

- A population-based study followed 438 middle-aged Australian-born women for 6 years, tracking their life satisfaction and attitudes toward menopause and aging as they moved through the menopausal transition. The study found that life satisfaction was positively correlated with feelings toward the partner and exercise. That is, the better they felt about their partners and the more they exercised, the more satisfied the women were with their lives.[37]

- Hoping to measure the effects of stress on mood, Australian researchers gave questionnaires to long-term exercisers, short-term exercisers, and nonexercisers. They found that, compared to the nonexercisers and short-term exercisers, the long-term exercisers were more positive in their thinking and felt more positive about their day-to-day experiences.[38]

- A study of the effects of aerobic exercise on pre- and postmenopausal women found significant enhancements in mood and reductions in somatic and vasomotor symptoms (hot flashes) immediately after an aerobics class. The researchers also found that when compared to nonexercisers, the exercisers had significantly more positive moods.[39]

Lifestyle Changes

Stop Smoking

Cigarettes contain nicotine, which speeds up the heart rate and can increase anxiety or nervousness. Although stopping is guaranteed to *raise* your anxiety levels for a while, you'll be better off in the long run.

Relax

Eliciting the relaxation response, a deliberate quieting of the body and mind that results in reduced heart and breathing rates, relaxed muscles, and lower levels of stress hormones, is one of the best ways of dealing with depression, anxiety, or irritability. (See "Relax" under "Lifestyle Changes" section in Chapter 7, page 143.) Practicing the relaxation response on a regular basis can help you manage the emotional changes associated with menopause, and may even be able to stop an emotional overreaction that's already in progress.

- An article appearing in the *American Journal of Psychiatry* described what happened when 22 volunteers suffering from generalized anxiety disorder or panic disorder were put on a relaxation and stress-reduction program. The anxiety and depression scores for 20 of the 22 participants dropped as a result of the meditation-based program, leading the researchers to conclude that meditation training can reduce symptoms in people suffering from anxiety disorder and related conditions.[40]
- Researchers at Harvard Medical School studying 33 postmenopausal women found that daily elicitation of the relaxation response significantly reduced not only hot flash intensity but also tension, anxiety and depression.[41]

Rising Stars?

Natural Progesterone

Many women have found that natural progesterone can help "smooth down" their moods. That's because progesterone stabilizes blood sugar levels, acts as a natural antidepressant, relieves anxiety, and helps you sleep, among other things.[42] When you don't have enough progesterone to counterbalance your estrogen, your body will be in a state of estrogen dominance and you'll most likely be moody, bloated, irritable and sleepless.

Don't expect the same good effects from synthetic progesterone (progestins), though. They can actually increase depression and destabilize blood sugar levels.[43]

Chapter Nine

What Happened to My Memory?

Have you noticed a slight slowing in brain activity since you turned 40? I certainly have. Before 40, I could call up facts and trivia in the time it took to snap my fingers. But now, I can almost feel the information grinding upward from the core of my brain, like a bubble rising through mud. And sometimes the bubble doesn't quite make it to the surface. (Who *was* the guy who played the lead in *My Cousin Vinny*, anyway?) Women going through menopause often experience some decline in memory since estrogen plays a part in brain function. Estrogen helps increase the supply of glucose and oxygen to the brain, enhances both memory and attention, promotes nerve growth, and protects brain cells against the effects of inflammation and oxidation. So when levels of this important hormone start to fall off, language skills, mood, memory, and ability to pay attention may also wane.

While these are normal age-related mental changes, dementia or Alzheimer's disease are not. Dementia involves a regression in memory, focus, thinking, and judgment that's severe enough to interfere with normal daily activities and social relationships. The most common cause of dementia is Alzheimer's disease, a progressive, irreversible decline in memory, language skills, orientation in time and space, and the ability to perform routine tasks. The hallmarks of Alzheimer's disease are *plaques* and *tangles*—deposits of plaque on the outer layers of the nerve cells in the brain, and tangled fibers inside the cells. Eventually the nerve cells deteriorate, fail to connect with other nerve cells, and die.

Besides Alzheimer's disease, the causes of dementia include Parkinson's disease, AIDS, Huntington's disease, a series of small strokes, and impaired blood flow to the brain (*vascular dementia*). Vascular dementia is primarily caused by uncontrolled high blood pressure, although elevated cholesterol, diabetes, and high levels of homocysteine in the blood can also be to blame.

The Problem

Estrogen plays an important part in memory and attention by increasing the supply of glucose and oxygen to the brain, promoting nerve growth and protecting brain cells against oxidation and inflammation. When estrogen levels decline at menopause, some women experience memory problems, trouble finding words, a loss of concentration, and "foggy thinking." These are normal signs of aging, not signs of dementia.

Why Does Cognitive Function Decline As We Age?

Memory problems, trouble thinking clearly, and difficulty in paying attention may be the result of one or more of the following:

- *Estrogen deficiency*—There are many regions of the brain (including those involved in memory) that have estrogen "docking sites," places where estrogen "plugs in" and activates brain tissue. Estrogen increases blood flow to the brain, raises the levels of brain neurotransmitters, and helps brain cells connect so they can send messages more efficiently. It also stimulates growth of the brain cells, particularly in the cerebral cortex and hypothalamus, and produces important enzymes that are key to the health of nerve cells. And brain cells are protected against the effects of inflammation and oxidation, thanks to estrogen. Too little estrogen brings about the opposite.
- *Depression*—Depression has long been known to impair mental function. The fatigue, brooding, negative thinking, changes in eating habits, and crying that often accompany depression can make it all but impossible for a person to focus on anything outside of herself.
- *Hormonal imbalances*—Estrogen and progesterone aren't the only hormones that decline with age. Other brain hormones also fall, including DHEA, melatonin, and pregnenolone, although the effects that these reductions may have on the brain are still unknown.
- *Injury*—Trauma to the brain, whether from an obvious hit on the head or the subtle leaking of blood into tissues surrounding the brain, can certainly affect brain function.
- *Neurologic disease*—Various diseases of the brain/nervous system, such as multiple sclerosis or ALS, can play a role in mental impairment.
- *Nutrient deficiencies*—A healthy brain requires a good supply of a variety of nutrients, from B-

vitamins to essential fatty acids. A deficiency in any of these substances may be partially to blame for reduced brain function.

- *Oxidative stress*—Oxidation and free radical damage can overwhelm the body's defenses through exposure to cigarette smoke, alcohol, pollution, chemicals, or high levels of stress. Free radical damage to the brain can impair mental function.
- *Oxygen starvation*—As circulation to the brain slows due to clogged arteries, a lack of exercise, smoking, or other factors, brain cells can "suffocate" and die.
- *Stroke*—Areas of the brain that are deprived of the nutrients and oxygen supplied by the blood will become damaged and may die. While the effects of a large stroke will be obvious, cumulative damage caused by strokes that are small enough to pass unnoticed can cause a decline in cognitive function.

Does Estrogen Replacement Counteract Mental Changes?

Although the impact of estrogen on mental function has been studied for more than 50 years, the verdict is still out. While one review of 17 randomized, controlled studies found that hormone replacement therapy helped improve verbal memory in some patients (particularly if the patient suffered from other menopausal symptoms),[1] the HERS study of 1,063 older postmenopausal women with heart disease found that 4 years of hormone therapy didn't result in better cognitive function.[2]

As for the role of estrogen in warding off Alzheimer's disease, a 2001 cohort study involving 280 postmenopausal women found that using estrogen did *not* reduce the risk of Alzheimer's.[3] Nor did it appear to slow the progression of the disease.[4]

In General, You Want To:

- keep your brain active
- keep your brain well-nourished
- keep your brain arteries in shape by controlling blood pressure, cholesterol, diabetes, etc.

What You Can Do About it

Vitamins and Phytochemicals

Antioxidants

Low blood levels of antioxidants have been associated with cognitive deficits, including Alzheimer's disease. While not all the studies agree, it seems clear that a lack of beta-carotene and vitamins C and E in the diet and/or the blood is connected to poorer cognitive function. Consider these studies:

Antioxidants in General

- The link between antioxidant consumption and cognitive function was examined in 260 elderly Spaniards. The volunteers did not have significant cognitive problems. The ones who scored higher on tests measuring cognitive function also consumed more beta-carotene, vitamin C, and vitamin E, as well as fiber, folate, zinc, iron, and carbohydrate.[5]

Beta-Carotene

- In one population-based study, Dutch researchers studied more than 5,000 people ages 55–95 and found that those who had a low intake of beta-carotene were more likely to have cognitive difficulties.[6]
- British researchers studied 251 people suffering from Alzheimer's disease, Parkinson's disease, and various other forms of dementia, as well as healthy volunteers. The researchers found that those suffering from vascular dementia had low blood levels of beta-carotene.[7]

Vitamin C

- A look at 921 Britons, age 65 and older, found that those with a lower vitamin C intake and lower blood levels of this vitamin were more likely to suffer from cognitive damage.[8]

Vitamin C and Beta-Carotene

- Of 442 seniors in Switzerland, those with greater levels of vitamin C and beta-carotene in their blood did better on tests of recall, recognition, and vocabulary.[9]

Vitamin E

- One of the most recent studies, published in 2002 in the *Archives of Neurology*, looked at 2,889 men and women, age 65 to 102. The participants were divided into five groups, depending upon how much vitamin E they consumed. While cognitive function declined in all groups over time, the decline was 36 percent slower in those in the highest vitamin E group, compared to the lowest.[10]

- A 2002 study appearing in the *Journal of the American Medical Association* looked at 815 people age 65 and older who did not have Alzheimer's disease. The participants were watched for an average of approximately 4 years, and their food intake was noted. The researchers found that those who consumed more vitamin E from foods had a lower risk of developing Alzheimer's disease.[11]

Vitamins C and E

- American researchers followed 633 seniors for an average of 4.3 years. All were disease free at the beginning of the study, and 91 developed Alzheimer's by study's end. None of the 50 people who were taking vitamin C or E supplements developed the disease, although researchers expected to see at least 2 or 3 new cases among them.[12]

Caution: See the cautions for these vitamins in Chapter 4.

Recommendation: There is no established dosage of vitamin E for prevention or treatment of dementia; however, some experts recommend daily doses of up to 2,000 IU of vitamin E, 1,000 mg of vitamin C, and 25,000 IU (15 mg) of beta-carotene.

Antioxidants As an Alzheimer's Remedy?

It appears that maintaining moderate to high levels of antioxidants in the blood could help ward off cognitive problems. But here comes the $64,000 question:

Will giving antioxidants to people who already have memory problems (i.e., Alzheimer's patients) improve their mental performance? Although there isn't much research that addresses this question, there is some:

- A large-scale, double-blind study looked at the effect of vitamin E and a drug called selegiline (designed to improve cognitive performance) on 341 people suffering from moderate Alzheimer's disease. The participants were given either 2,000 IU of vitamin E per day, selegiline, both, or a placebo. Then the patients were observed for the next 2 years to see who would suffer a "bad outcome" (defined as losing the ability to perform the tasks of daily living, developing dementia, requiring institutionalization, or dying). When the treatments were compared to the placebo, the researchers found that taking vitamin E reduced the risk of a "bad outcome" by 53 percent, the drug reduced it by 43 percent, and the combination reduced it by 31 percent. Plus, it took 230 days longer for the "bad outcome" to appear in those taking the vitamin E (versus the placebo), 215 days longer in those taking the drug, and 145 days longer in those taking both.[13] The Alzheimer's Association commented on this study: "Vitamin E worked at least as well as selegiline on Alzheimer's progression in this study and had fewer side effects. Vitamin E also costs less. For these reasons it is preferred over selegiline in Alzheimer's disease treatment. Vitamin E is considered to be a 'benign' medication and most people can take it without side effects."[14]
- The American Psychiatric Association also took

note of vitamin E. In their 1997 "Practice Guideline for the Treatment of Patients with Alzheimer's Disease and Other Dementias of Late Life," the organization suggested that vitamin E can help "delay progression of Alzheimer's disease" in patients with mild or moderate impairment.[15]

- In 2001, the American Academy of Neurology examined the medical literature and published guidelines for doctors dealing with dementia. In their report, they stated that vitamin E most likely slowed the worsening of symptoms.[16]

- Finally, a study appearing in the *Journal of the American Medical Association* in June 2002 suggested that "a diet rich in foods containing vitamin E may help protect some people against Alzheimer's disease."[17]

We don't know nearly enough yet to make definitive statements on the antioxidant-dementia connection. More study needs to be done, but it looks as if good amounts of fresh fruits, vegetables, and other foods containing beta-carotene, vitamin C, vitamin E, and other antioxidants, as well as the judicious use of supplements, could be beneficial.

Ginkgo Biloba Extract

Taken from the world's oldest living tree (it's been around some 200 million years!), ginkgo biloba extract is a popular remedy for circulation problems and cognitive decline. It's also been promoted as an effective aid for improving dementia and mental function, due to its ability to improve circulation to the brain. Ginkgo is also believed to have antioxidant effects, protect cell walls, regulate the workings of certain neurotransmitters, and otherwise help keep the brain working smoothly.

Ginkgo and Age-Related Mental Changes

Let's first look at some of the studies involving the use of ginkgo biloba by seniors who did *not* have Alzheimer's or other forms of dementia:

- A study of the effects of ginkgo on daily living and mood followed 5,028 senior citizens with an average age of 69. Over a 4-month period, 1,000 of them took 120 mg of a ginkgo extract every day; the rest took a placebo. Those taking the ginkgo performed better on tests measuring their ability to handle daily activities and reported more positive changes in their sleeping patterns and mood.[18]

- In one study, 260 dementia-free male and female volunteers age 60 and older were given either 180 mg of a ginkgo biloba extract daily or a placebo. At the end of the 6-week treatment period, the researchers looked at the results of various neuropsychological tests and concluded that the ginkgo extract improved memory processing.[19]

Ginkgo and Alzheimer's Disease

Now let's look at ginkgo's effects on people who were already suffering from Alzheimer's disease or other forms of dementia:

- For a year-long, double-blind study, participants were given either 120 mg of a ginkgo extract daily or a placebo. The results of the study showed that ginkgo aided in cognitive performance and social functioning in people with mild or moderately severe Alzheimer's. For those who began the study with mild dementia, the ginkgo triggered improvement. For those who began with moderate dementia, the ginkgo helped slow the decline.[20]

- From the *Journal of the American Medical Association* comes this 1997 study of 202 people suffering from mild to moderate Alzheimer's or stroke-induced dementia. The patients were given either 120 mg per day of a ginkgo extract or a placebo. One year later, the findings indicated that the ginkgo extract stabilized and, in some cases, improved the social and cognitive functioning of those already suffering from dementia—and that the results lasted for 6–12 months. Ginkgo's helpful effects were modest, but measurable.[21]

- Dr. Le Bars of the New York University Medical Center, who conducted several studies on ginkgo biloba and dementia, published a review of the medical literature in 2000. In his paper, he noted that ginkgo biloba extract worked better in those who already had dementia than in healthy people, and that benefits could be seen more clearly when one looked at broad measures of cognitive ability, rather than the results of simple memory tests used in some studies. He also stated that while we haven't yet established the most effective dose of ginkgo, 240 mg per day appears to produce a good effect.[22]

- The noted Cochrane Reviews also reviewed the scientific literature, presenting their findings in 2002. The review concluded that "overall, there is promising evidence of improvement in cognition and function associated with ginkgo," and that "ginkgo biloba appears to be safe in use with no excess side effects compared to placebo."[23]

As is the case with vitamin E, we can't make conclusive statements about ginkgo biloba since we don't have enough high-quality, large-scale studies to say that it absolutely does or does not work. However, the weight of mounting evidence strongly suggests that ginkgo biloba can help those with mild to moderate Alzheimer's disease, and certain other forms of dementia.

Caution: Although ginkgo is generally considered to be safe, it can trigger problems in sensitive people or if used inappropriately:

- Potential side effects include headaches, dizziness, palpitations, allergic skin reactions and mild gastrointestinal upset.
- Ginkgo thins the blood, so using it along with blood-thinning medications (including aspirin) may cause problems. Do not take ginkgo if you have a bleeding disorder.
- Ginkgo may increase blood pressure if taken along with thiazide diuretics.

Recommendation: There is no established dosage of ginkgo biloba. For Alzheimer's or other forms of dementia, a typical dosage is 120–240 mg per day, divided into two or three doses.

Rising Stars?

Here are some approaches that may prove valuable when more research with human subjects is conducted:

- *Exercise for the brain*—If you enjoy reading, doing crossword puzzles, going to museums, traveling, or following the news, keep it up. A recent study appearing in the *Journal of the American Medical Association* tracked 801 older Catholic priests, nuns, and brothers for an average of 4.5 years each, all of them dementia-free when the study began. The researchers found that those who frequently participated in brain-stimulating activities had a reduced risk of developing Alzheimer's disease.[24]
- *B vitamins*—A study backed by the National Institute on Aging found that elevated levels of an amino acid called homocysteine in the blood could nearly double the odds of developing Alzheimer's disease. For 8 years, researchers followed 1,092 people, of average age 76 and free of dementia at the beginning of the study. When the researchers compared those who eventually developed dementia or Alzheimer's to those who did not, they found that those who had larger amounts of homocysteine in their blood at the beginning of the study were more likely to develop problems.[25] Neil Buckholtz, Ph.D., chief of the Dementias of Aging program at the National Institute on Aging, noted that "the evidence is beginning to mount regarding homocysteine's role in dementia."[26] What's the link to B-vitamins? You can lower the amount of homocysteine in your blood by taking vitamin B_6, B_{12}, and folic acid. (See recommendations for each of these vitamins in Chapter 4.)
- *Acetyl-L-carnitine*—A natural substance similar to the brain chemical acetylcholine in structure, acetyl-L-carnitine was used in a Stanford University study on 334 patients with probable Alz-

heimer's. Acetyl-L-carnitine was found to slow the progression of the disease in the younger patients (60 years old or younger).[27] Typical doses range between 1,500 and 3,000 mg per day.

- *Phosphatidylserine*—A phospholipid found in concentrated amounts in the brain, phosphatidylserine (PS) helps regulate the brain chemicals that carry messages between the neurons. Although study results have been mixed, taking 100 mg of PS three times a day may encourage mild improvement in cognitive function,[28] and no side effects are apparent at this dosage.

- *Vinpocetine*—Vinpocetine, like ginkgo, increases the blood supply to the brain and stimulates the brain's uptake of glucose. It may also increase the production of brain chemicals that ferry messages between the neurons.[29] In a study involving 12 healthy female volunteers, taking 40 mg of vinpocetine for just 3 days improved memory significantly.[30] Typical dosage is 15 mg per day, divided into three doses.

- *Glucose*—Finally someone is telling you to add sugar to your diet! Glucose is the brain's fuel, and increasing its supply may improve your memory almost instantly. One study of 28 healthy seniors (average age 73) found that giving 50 grams of glucose (about 3½ T sugar) enhanced recall, verbal fluency, figural fluency, and performance on a test of divided attention, compared to those given saccharin.[31] Another researcher found that increasing blood glucose levels improved memory by 100 percent in some Alzheimer's patients.[32] If you eat sugar by itself, it takes 15–30 minutes to be released into the bloodstream. If you take it in conjunction with fat, protein, or complex carbohydrates, it will take longer—up to an hour. Since blood sugar ups and downs can exacerbate other conditions (i.e., diabetes, depression, anxiety, irritability, etc.), you may want to eat something sugary as part of a meal about an hour before you need to be especially sharp.

Chapter Ten

The Wonderful, All-Weather Vagina

The vagina is a fantastic organ. Accommodating, resilient, and self-cleaning to boot, its lining is thickened and toughened to withstand the rigors of sexual intercourse, thanks to the influence of estrogen. But estrogen's role doesn't stop there. It also increases the production of a type of sugar present in the vaginal tract called *glycogen*. Friendly bacteria called *Lactobacillus acidophilus* (the same kind you find in yogurt) that feed on the glycogen produce acid, creating an acidic environment in the vagina that keeps "bad" bacteria and yeasts from flourishing. A rich blood supply keeps the vagina moist and produces lubricating secretions during sexual arousal. All in all, it's a hospitable place for the male organ to visit, a sanitary passageway leading from the outside of the body to the uterus, and a pliable birth canal that can accommodate the passage of a full term infant, if necessary.

But when estrogen levels decline, many of these

benefits start to wane. The vagina itself begins to shrink and atrophy. The vaginal lining thins, becoming more fragile, less elastic, and more likely to become injured during intercourse. And as blood flow to the genitals decreases, vaginal lubrication diminishes, causing dryness that may make intercourse difficult. Even clitoral stimulation can become irritating. To top it off, vaginal infections may make more appearances than ever before. Some women lose interest in sex after menopause, but many experts believe that this has more to do with a smorgasbord of vaginal/urinary symptoms than with the decline of the female hormones themselves. The three biggest vaginal difficulties associated with menopause are dryness, infections, and a lack of interest in sex.

The Problem—Vaginal Dryness

A decline in estrogen causes the walls of the vagina to thin, become drier, and grow less elastic, and the blood supply to the organ decreases. Vaginal dryness and painful intercourse can result.

While millions of American women of all ages suffer from vaginal dryness, those who are postmenopausal (particularly those who have experienced surgical menopause) are the most likely to be confronted with this problem. The signs are hard to miss: Your vagina feels dry; you're just not lubricating like you used to; and intercourse becomes uncomfortable, difficult, or irritating. You may also feel a burning or itching sensation and experience vaginal bleeding after intercourse.

In General, You Want To:

- keep it lubricated
- keep the tissues moist from within
- keep it irritant-free
- keep it toned

What You Can Do About it

There are several dietary and lifestyle changes you can incorporate to prevent or ease vaginal dryness.

Diet

Your basic dietary strategy for warding off vaginal dryness should be to keep your tissues well-hydrated and avoid substances that tend to dry them out.

- *Drink plenty of water*—Drink a minimum of 8 glasses of water per day to increase the level of your bodily fluids and keep your tissues well moisturized.
- *Avoid alcoholic beverages*—Any way you look at it, alcohol is drying to your tissues.
- *Stay away from caffeine*—Caffeine is another substance that can sap moisture. Limit your intake of caffeinated beverages to one per day and watch out for drugs that contain caffeine. (See the "Take Care With Caffeine" section in Chapter 5, page 86.)

Lifestyle Changes

A trio of lifestyle changes offers the best relief from vaginal dryness: Avoid substances that can irritate or dry delicate vaginal tissues, use lubricants or moisturizers, and keep the vagina in good shape.

Avoid Substances That Are Drying or Irritating

First of all, don't douche—your vagina is self-cleaning, so douching is unnecessary. And hosing it down with water, vinegar-water, or manufactured preparations will simply wash away your natural lubricants. Stay away from deodorant soaps, bubble baths, or feminine deodorants, all of which can dry or irritate vaginal tissues. Also, watch out for medications that can "dry you out," including antihistamines, antibiotics, antidepressants, anything containing caffeine, decongestants, diuretics, hypertension medication, narcotics, sedatives, or tranquilizers. Finally, be aware that radiation therapy or chemotherapy can dry out vaginal tissues. Consult your physician for help in this case.

Use Lubricants or Moisturizers

Your own natural secretions are the best lubricant, and you may find that they are sufficient if you extend the length of time you spend in foreplay. If not, try using a water-based lubricant like K-Y Jelly or Astroglide or a vitamin E ointment or suppositories just prior to intercourse. But don't lubricate with oil-based products like petroleum jelly, baby oil or cocoa butter, as they can coat the vaginal lining and block your own natural secretions. They can also weaken latex condoms and allow small holes to develop.

Special, low pH moisturizers that are available over the counter can help the vagina rebuild a moist, protective layer while maintaining its crucial infection-fighting acidic environment. A vaginal suppository called Replens moisturizes for up to three days, while simultaneously helping fight vaginal infections.

Keep the Vagina in Good Shape

Have regular sexual workouts. Just as your leg muscles get stronger when you jog regularly and atrophy when they're ignored, your vagina benefits from regular workouts. Intercourse and/or manual stimulation will increase the flow of blood to the area, stimulate the lubricating glands, and promote vaginal elasticity. Intercourse also maintains vaginal tone, and women who have sexual relations three or more times a month tend to have less vaginal atrophy.[1]

You may also want to consider applying estrogen in cream form directly to vaginal tissues. Although this book is designed to help you discover nondrug approaches to managing menopausal symptoms, this treatment is worth mentioning because of its superior ability to restore vaginal and bladder health and function. While other methods of dealing with vaginal and urinary changes mainly ease the symptoms, this can actually *reverse* vaginal dryness, atrophy and the thinning and inflammation of vaginal tissues.[2]

Although some of the estrogen is eventually absorbed into your bloodstream, the levels are usually extremely low (particularly when the cream is in the form of *estriol*, a weaker estrogen). The effects of the estrogen cream appear to be confined to the vagina and urinary tract alone, so it doesn't carry the risks of standard estrogen therapy. In fact, so little estrogen is released into the bloodstream that taking progesterone to counteract overgrowth of the uterine lining is not needed for short-term use (less than 8 months).[3]

Another method of vaginal administration of estrogen is the estrogen-releasing vaginal ring. Positioned in the vagina for 3 months at a time, the ring releases tiny amounts of estrogen that revive both your vaginal lining and your lubricating abilities. If you're having a terrible time with vaginal dryness or other vaginal problems, you may want to talk to your physician about trying an estrogen cream or a vaginal ring.

The Problem—Vaginal Infections

The vagina's natural acidic environment becomes more alkaline as estrogen levels drop, making it more prone to infections. As the estrogen-dependent glycogen supply in vaginal tissues decreases, friendly bacteria have less to feed on and produce less acid. This less acidic, more alkaline environment is much more hospitable to *E. coli* bacteria and yeasts, which are common causes of vaginal infections.

Vaginal discharge is the most common symptom of a vaginal infection, often accompanied by itching, burning and odor. Most vaginal infections respond well to treatment with antibiotic, antiviral or antifungal medications. Antifungal medications (e.g., Gyne-Lotrimin, Monistat, etc.) are the only kind that you can buy over the counter, and they are designed solely for the purpose of treating yeast infections. So if you have another kind of infection, you're not sure, or you have recurring infections, see your health care provider for treatment.

In General, You Want To:

- keep it clean
- keep it dry
- keep it acidic
- keep invading organisms hungry
- keep your vitamin C levels up

What You Can Do About It

The best way to prevent a vaginal infection is to maintain a healthy vaginal environment.

Diet

Believe it or not, what you eat can affect the health of your vagina.

Keep Invading Organisms Hungry

Sugar promotes the growth of yeast, a major promoter of vaginal infections, so try to keep your intake of high sugar foods to a minimum.

Foods, Phytochemicals, Vitamins, and Minerals

Foods that increase vaginal acidity also help fight infections.

Keep It Acidic

The acid produced by lactobacilli is necessary to keep bacteria and yeasts at bay, so eat more yogurt! (Make sure it contains live cultures of *Lactobacillus acidophilus* and it's sugar-free, since sugar promotes the growth of yeast.)

Keep Your Vitamin C Levels Up

Vitamin C (ascorbic acid) makes your urine more acidic, which will help ward off bacteria.

Lifestyle Changes

Keep It Clean

Wash the genital area regularly and be sure to clean inside the folds to remove bacteria. When you use the toilet, wipe from front to back so that germs from the anal area aren't swept into the vagina.

Keep It Dry

Sitting around in wet underwear or a wet bathing suit promotes the growth of yeast and bacteria, so wear underwear with an absorbent cotton crotch, consider using minipads if you have significant discharge, change into something dry as soon as you finish swimming, and get out of wet, sweaty workout clothes and underwear right after a workout. Also, don't wear tight-fitting pants, panty hose, girdles, or other clothes that restrict the flow of air to the crotch area and increase heat and moisture retention.

Keep It Irritant-Free

Irritants promote vaginal infections, so don't use perfumed or deodorant soaps, bubble bath, bath oil, or perfumed feminine products (e.g., hygiene sprays and scented pads and tampons). Don't douche. Glycerin-based soaps are preferable. After swimming, be sure to shower immediately to remove chlorine or seawater.

Increase Vaginal Acidity

To prevent yeast infections and help with lubrication, try inserting 1–2 Lactobacillus acidophilus capsules vaginally 4–6 hours before having intercourse. Or insert a tablespoon of plain yogurt vaginally with a tampon, then lie down for 10 minutes to let it "take."

Avoid taking antibiotics except when treating a bacterial infection, and even then only when it's absolutely necessary. (They don't help with viral infections and will kill your friendly bacteria for no reason.)

Finally, stay out of chlorinated swimming pools and hot tubs since they can make the vagina more alkaline and less acidic.

Keep It Lubricated

Don't have intercourse until you're really ready. Use a lubricant or moisturizer if necessary.

The Problem—Diminished Sex Drive

Some women experience a decline in sexual appetite, which is probably due to vaginal dryness, difficulty with intercourse and increased infections, rather than a decline in hormone levels.

The thinning and drying of vaginal tissues, coupled with a decrease in blood flow to the genitals and an increase in vaginal infections, can really put a damper on your sex life.

In General, You Want To:

- keep it irritant-free
- keep it lubricated
- keep it toned

What You Can Do About It

There are lots of books on the market that are loaded with creative ideas for spicing up your sex life, and it may pay to invest in a few. Here are two ideas that you might not want to overlook:

Exercise

Kegel Exercises

Lack of muscle tone may be another reason your interest in sex can wane. First introduced over 40 years ago, Kegel exercises are designed to strengthen the muscle that runs from your pubic bone to your tail bone—the pubococcygeus or PC muscle. This muscle provides much-needed support for your internal pelvic organs and vaginal tissues, and keeping it strong can improve sexual satisfaction (for both you and your partner), and help you improve your bladder control. You can access this muscle the next time you urinate by stopping the flow in midstream. Try to stop the flow at least two or three times each time you urinate. The muscle you contract to accomplish this is your PC muscle.

You can contract your PC muscle anywhere, anytime, and no one will know you're doing it. Begin by holding it for 3 seconds, then relaxing for 3 seconds; repeat 10 times. Eventually, you should hold for up to 10 seconds at a time. You can also contract and relax the PC muscle as fast as you can 10 times in a row. Gradually increase until you can do it 50 times in a row.

Lifestyle Changes

The EROS-Clitoral Therapy Device

Along with intercourse difficulties and increased infections, an important cause of diminished sexual arousal is a decrease in blood flow to the genitals. This handheld gadget creates a gentle vacuum over the clitoris that helps enhance arousal. A study of 20 women reported in 2001[4] found that the device increased blood flow to the clitoris, improved vaginal lubrication, increased orgasmic ability and enhanced overall sexual satisfaction. If you're interested, ask your health care provider about getting a prescription.

Rising Stars?

There are no vitamins or other supplements supported by the scientific literature as helpful for easing vaginal changes. However, here's one "rising star" that has made a promising start:

- *Soy isoflavones*—One study found that postmenopausal women who consumed the equivalent of about 200 mg of isoflavones daily showed signs of estrogenic activity, including higher numbers of cells lining the vaginal wall, which can help ease vaginal dryness and irritation.[5] In another study, postmenopausal women received 10 percent of their energy intake in the form of one of three phytoestrogenic plants: soybean flour, red clover sprouts, or linseed. After 6 weeks, vaginal cell maturation (the thickening and toughening of cells lining the vagina) increased significantly.[6] To ease vaginal dryness and irritation, consume up to 150 mg of soy isoflavones daily. Although this study used 200 mg of soy isoflavones, this is not recommended. (See cautions, page 59, in "Soy or Soybeans" section in Chapter 4.)

Chapter Eleven

Quick, Where's the Bathroom?

Like most of us, you've probably taken your ability to urinate (and not) absolutely for granted. And then one day the problems start. There's *urinary urgency*, the feeling that you have to go right now; *urinary frequency*, the need to go more frequently; *nocturia*, the need to go several times a night; and *incontinence*, the inability to *keep* from going, whether it's convenient or not.

Incontinence can be further broken down into the following:

- *stress incontinence*—uncontrolled loss of urine when coughing, sneezing, lifting heavy objects, or doing anything else that increases pressure inside the abdomen
- *urge incontinence*—the urgent need to void the bladder, followed by an uncontrolled loss of urine
- *total incontinence*—constant loss of urine due to a urinary sphincter that doesn't close completely

Although urinary problems can be caused by lots of different conditions, many of them can be traced to the atrophy of the urethra and bladder, brought on by the lack of estrogen. For many postmenopausal women, the urine "reservoir" (the bladder) and the "dam" (the urinary sphincter) that used to hold the urine in place simply aren't up to the job anymore.

Like the vagina, the bladder is studded with estrogen receptors and depends upon this hormone to help maintain its function, muscle tone, and resilience. A decline in estrogen affects the bladder in ways similar to those seen in the vagina. Both the urethra (the tube that carries the urine from the bladder to the outside of the body) and the lining of the bladder thin and lose muscle tone, making them less able to retain the urine. Incontinence is surprisingly common among women over 60, with at least 40 percent of them complaining about this condition.[1] The sagging of a portion of the bladder can cause urine to pool and be retained in the bladder, so that it never gets completely emptied. This leads to recurrent urinary tract infections, a condition that is two to three times more common in older women.[2]

The Problem

A decline in estrogen causes a loss of tissue, tone and function in the bladder and urethra, causing symptoms such as urinary urgency, incontinence and recurring bladder infections.

The Estrogen-Urinary Tract Connection

The postmenopausal lack of estrogen can result in:

- *Atrophy of urethra*—The urethra becomes weakened after menopause due to the loss of much of its collagen. The sphincter muscle that connects the bladder to the urethra loosens up, making it difficult to retain urine. Also, your sensitivity to urine in the bladder increases, making you feel the need to go to the bathroom more often.

- *Poor bladder tone*—The bladder is designed to contract and push urine out once the sphincter muscle relaxes. But without estrogen, the bladder becomes weak and flabby, doesn't contract well, and does a less efficient job of expelling the urine.

- *Bladder prolapse*—A weakened, poorly toned bladder is more susceptible to prolapse, a condition in which one part of the organ sags. Urine that collects in the base of the sagging portion may simply stay in the bladder. This can cause infections and a feeling of urinary urgency, even after you've just urinated.

- *Increased infections*—Urine that doesn't get eliminated provides a prime medium for bacterial infection. The vagina can also contribute to bladder infections since their openings are only about an inch apart. When the vagina's pH becomes more alkaline, discouraging the growth of friendly bacteria, more "bad" bacteria flourish near the urethra. It's not hard to imagine how infectious organisms could take the short walk from the vagina to the urethra and continue on up to the bladder. Not surprisingly, recurring urinary tract infections are a big problem in older women, affecting as many as 30 percent of women over the age of 80.[3]

In General, You Want To:

- empty your bladder regularly and completely
- tone up your PC muscle

- drink plenty of water
- avoid smoking, caffeine, or medications that cause urinary problems

What You Can Do About It—Urinary Urgency or Incontinence

Many women can regain bladder control by using a few simple techniques:

Diet

Drink 6–8 Glasses of Water a Day

While you might think this is the last thing you should do for incontinence, your bladder can become irritated if your urine is too concentrated. Keeping it diluted by drinking lots of water can help.

Watch Your Caffeine Intake

Caffeine is known to increase urinary difficulties. Keep your consumption down to one caffeinated drink per day and monitor your intake of caffeine-containing medications.

Exercise

Strengthen Your PC Muscle

The best thing you can do to prevent incontinence or regain control is to make sure your PC muscle is in great shape. This muscle provides much-needed support for your internal pelvic organs and is responsible for stopping the flow of urine. If it's weak, you can find yourself leaking urine. Do your Kegel exercises regularly to keep your muscles strong. (See Kegel exercises, page 196, in Chapter 10.)

Strengthen Your Abdominals

All of the muscles in your abdominal area should be kept strong and toned to maintain the health and strength of your pelvic region. If your pelvic area is weak, organs can sag and put pressure on your bladder. Get plenty of exercise involving the lower body (jogging, cycling, dancing, etc.). Do sit-ups, leg lifts, and other abdominal strengtheners on a regular basis.

Lifestyle Changes

Avoid Triggers

Smoking, antidepressants, antihistamines and diuretics are all known to increase urinary difficulties. If you're currently taking any medications, ask your physician if they may be related to urinary problems. If so, see if you can switch to something different.

Urinate Every 2–3 Hours

Make it a point to visit the bathroom on a regular basis—don't wait until you're desperate! This will keep your bladder fairly empty, which is good for controlling incontinence and preventing infections.

Wait a Minute!

Your bladder may not be completely empty after you've urinated, which could be a reason you'll soon feel the urge to go again. Wait several seconds after you've finished urinating to see if you can get rid of any residual urine.

What You Can Do About It—Urinary Tract Infections

If you've got a urinary tract infection (UTI), you'll soon know it. The symptoms include pain or burning upon urination, a strong urge to urinate although only a little urine is passed, frequent urination, pressure in your lower abdomen, itching, and possibly a fever. Taking an antibacterial medication will probably get rid of the infection quickly, but if you tend to suffer from recurrent infections, you need to watch what you're doing.

Since UTIs often originate as vaginal infections, review the tips for prevention in the "The Problem—Vaginal Infections" section, page 192, in Chapter 10. Then, try these:

Diet

Drink 6–8 Glasses of Water a Day
Water dilutes urine and flushes bacteria out.

Cranberry Juice
Drinking unsweetened cranberry juice works! Recent research has made it clear that substances in cranberry juice make it difficult for bacteria to "stick" to the sides of the urinary tract. Unable to latch on to anything, the bacteria are simply swept out with the urine. You'll need to drink 1-2 cups a day to get the beneficial effects. But make sure you get the unsweetened kind because sugar increases bacterial growth.

- Back in 1994, a study published in the *Journal of the American Medical Association* looked at what happened when 153 elderly women were given either cranberry juice or a placebo drink every day.[4] The results suggested that cranberry juice could reduce the frequency of bacteriuria and pyuria (signs of urinary tract infections) in older women.

- More recently, Finnish researchers looked at the effects of a cranberry-lingonberry juice mixture in 150 women suffering from a urinary tract infection caused by *E. coli*. The women were asked to either take the cranberry-lingonberry drink, take a lactobacillus drink, or do nothing (the control group). After 6 months, there was a 20 percent reduction in recurrence of UTI in the cranberry drink group, compared to the control group. Those taking the lactobacillus drink actually had more UTIs than the control group.[5]

Lifestyle Changes

Urinate Right After Having Sexual Intercourse
This helps to flush out any bacteria that might have entered your urethra.

Empty Your Bladder Often
Urine that "stands" in the bladder for long periods of time tends to attract bacteria.

Try Vaginal Estrogen Cream
Applying estrogen (estradiol) in cream form directly to the vaginal area is a safe and effective treatment for genitourinary atrophy and recurrent UTI.[6] The loss of estrogen increases urinary urgency and atrophy of the bladder and the urethra, but using a little cream on or near the affected tissues may work wonders at restoring their func-

tion. A recent study of the effectiveness of vaginal estrogen cream plus Kegel exercises found that this combination could help ease postmenopausal stress incontinence in as little as three months.[7]

Chapter Twelve

To Sleep, Perchance to Dream

I was 44 years old when all of a sudden I forgot how to fall asleep. After a lifetime of dropping off the minute my head touched the pillow, I abruptly found myself tossing and turning for hours, night after night, praying for sleep to overtake me and put me out of my misery. Then, if I was lucky, sometime between 2 and 3 a.m. I'd drift into a very light sleep, thin as cheesecloth and unrefreshing as a hot shower on a 90-degree day. On other terrible nights, I never managed to drop off at all. I kept telling my husband, "I feel like I'm just not making any 'sleep juice' anymore—or whatever it is that used to make me fall asleep."

Insomnia (the inability to sleep) was my first and most troubling symptom of perimenopause. And although none of the doctors I consulted even asked about my menopausal status, insomnia is a common symptom accompanying "the change," affecting between one-third and one-half of menopausal women at one time or another. It comes in several forms:

- The first kind of insomnia is the inability to drop off to sleep once you're in bed and the lights are off. You toss, turn, count sheep, or do deep breathing exercises, and absolutely nothing happens.
- With the second kind, falling asleep is no problem, but you wake up in the middle of the night and then find yourself unable to go back to sleep. Women who experience hot flashes or night sweats or who have bladder problems often suffer from this kind of insomnia. This is the kind of insomnia most often seen in peri- and postmenopausal women.
- The third kind may not involve actual awakenings but an overall quality of sleep that is poor. Even when you've slept an adequate number of hours, you wake up feeling tired and unrefreshed.

But no matter what kind of insomnia you have, the bottom line is this: If you're not getting enough sleep, you're bound to be tired, irritable, and depressed the next day. And too many of these sleepless nights can seriously affect the quality of your life.

The Problem

Insomnia, the inability to fall asleep, stay asleep, or be refreshed by sleep, is a common complaint of women during the menopausal years. Hot flashes, night sweats, or bladder problems may disrupt sleep. Reduced sleep can lead to fatigue, irritability, and depression during the day.

The Sleep Zappers

Babies effortlessly sleep for up to 18 hours a day, and teenagers usually have no trouble sleeping soundly no matter how erratic their eating, exercise, or sleeping habits. But with age, "anti-sleep" changes occur, including altered hormone levels, body temperature fluctuations, and decreased levels of physical activity. As a result, you may tend to wake up more often during the night, and stay awake longer each time you do. Add to these physical changes the stresses of dealing with menopause, children, your spouse, finances, a job, and the insomnia itself, and good sleep can seem like a distant memory.

Sleep and Body Temperature

Your ability to fall asleep is very much related to your body temperature. While you might think that you maintain a steady 98.6 degrees inside, your temperature actually varies as much as a couple of degrees throughout the day and night. Your body temperature is at its lowest at about 4 a.m. and slowly starts to rise just before the sun comes up. During the day it continues climbing, dropping a bit in midafternoon, then rising to an all-time high at about 6 p.m. Shortly after that, your temperature begins to recede and continues to drop until about 4 a.m.

You tend to be most active and alert during the hours when your body temperature is at its highest (i.e., around midday and 6 p.m.) And you become least active and sleepiest when your temperature declines— in the midafternoon and in the very early morning hours (around 3:30 a.m.). Next time you feel like you can't keep your eyes open in the middle of the afternoon, blame it on a drop in body temperature.

The important thing to remember about all of this is that before you can fall asleep, your body temperature has to drop. Just think of how hard it is to sleep in a hot room on a summer's night. Your body temperature can't drop off fast enough or far enough to let you fall asleep. With this in mind, you can see how a hot flash would jolt you out of sleep and leave your mind and body ready for action. And even subtle rises in temperature, ones you might not even notice, can cause middle-of-the-night awakenings that can last as long as a couple of hours.

Body temperature has also been implicated in insomnia that's not related to menopause. Many chronic insomniacs just naturally have lower peak temperatures and higher low temperatures—that is, their temperatures fluctuate less than would be expected and may not fall low enough at night to bring on deep and lengthy sleep. The elderly can also have problems sleeping because their body temperatures not only fluctuate less but tend to rise and fall earlier in the day, making them more likely to fall asleep earlier, wake up earlier, and sleep less.

Erratic Blood Sugar Levels

Since your brain depends on a steady supply of glucose, a drop in blood sugar can send your brain into "crisis mode." The adrenal glands release adrenaline, which pushes blood glucose back up but also increases anxiety and wakefulness. If you eat sugary foods close to bedtime or you're on a strict diet that leaves you hungry, you may trigger a blood glucose rise and fall that can shake you out of a sound sleep.

Disruption of the Serotonin-Melatonin Cycle

Two brain chemicals, serotonin and melatonin, play important parts in regulating sleep. Serotonin wakes you up, makes you feel energetic, alert, and happy, while melatonin makes you feel drowsy and ready to sleep. Melatonin is actually converted from serotonin in response to exposure to light. When you're exposed to bright light, your brain makes serotonin; when the light goes dim, your brain converts the serotonin to melatonin. You've probably noticed this on short winter days when darkness falls early and you find yourself sleepy and longing for your bed at 5 p.m.

Traveling across time zones, working the midnight shift, changing work shifts, or living in a northerly area like Alaska where darkness lasts most of the day can seriously disrupt the serotonin-melatonin cycle. That's because a lack of regular exposure to dark and light can leave your body wondering when it's time to wake and to sleep.

Depression and Anxiety

Depression and anxiety are linked to insomnia as part of a vicious circle. While both are stressors that can contribute to sleeplessness, the lack of sleep is, itself, a stressor that can make depression and anxiety even worse. Take my word for it, you can get pretty anxious when you're staring at the clock at 4 a.m. and you've got to get up and go to work in three hours!

Progesterone deficiency, low blood sugar, alcohol ingestion, low levels of endorphins, and low serotonin levels can all contribute to depression and anxiety, which in turn can cause sleep disturbances.

Other Reasons for Insomnia

Some studies suggest that insomniacs have faster heart rates, faster brain wave patterns, and more muscle tension than normal sleepers do. Other reasons for poor sleep include:

- Alzheimer's disease or other forms of dementia
- allergies, asthma, or other breathing problems
- cigarette smoking
- disorders that make it necessary to urinate or have a bowel movement during the night
- emotional stress
- an environment that's not conducive to sleeping (e.g., too noisy, too hot, too cold, too much light, or a poor mattress or pillow)
- headaches
- heartburn, painful ulcers, or other gastrointestinal problems
- kidney disease
- pain due to illness, injury, or surgery

See your physician for help in handling these problems.

Certain medications and mood-altering substances can also disturb your sleep, including:

- alcohol
- antidepressants
- asthma medicines
- beta blockers and other medications for hypertension
- cocaine, amphetamines, marijuana, and other recreational drugs
- cortisone medications
- decongestants
- diet pills
- pain pills that contain caffeine
- steroids

Eliminating these substances or switching to different kinds of medication can make a big difference in the quality and duration of your sleep.

The Trouble with Sleeping Pills

The most obvious thing to do when you can't sleep well is to take some sort of sleeping medication, typically drugs that fall into the category of benzodiazepines (Valium, Xanax, Halcion, Klonopin, etc.). Sleeping pills are an easy fix that may work for a short time, but they're not the ultimate answer. While they will knock you out, they lessen deep sleep and REM (rapid eye movement or dream) sleep, so your sleep will be lighter and of poorer quality. They can also cause residual drowsiness, interactions with other drugs, and physical or psychological dependency. Finally, they do nothing to solve the underlying problem.

Over-the-counter sleeping aids (e.g., Tylenol PM and Excedrin PM) also have side effects, become less potent over time, and can be psychologically addicting. If you do decide to take a sleeping medication (either prescription or over-the-counter) for temporary sleep disturbances, use the smallest possible dose and do not take it for more than two weeks.

In General, You Want To:

- establish good sleeping habits
- create an environment conducive to sleep
- relax
- avoid stimulants or other substances that interfere with sleep

- encourage melatonin production
- exercise, but not too close to bedtime
- restore hormonal balance

What You Can Do About It

Diet

It's always wise to eat a nutritious, balanced diet, especially when you're feeling out of balance inside. Eating several small meals spaced throughout the day and a small bedtime snack can aid in digestion and help keep blood glucose levels on an even keel. But make sure you eat dinner several hours before bedtime, so you're not in the throes of heavy digestion when you're ready to turn in for the night.

Avoid Alcohol

Although a glass of wine or a beer around bedtime may seem like a good way to relax, 1 oz of alcohol within 2 hours of bedtime will disrupt the quality of your sleep, making it lighter, more fragmented, and more likely to produce early morning awakenings. It also suppresses deep sleep and dream sleep, and increases the tendency toward nightmares. Even worse, alcohol, a central nervous system depressant, can increase depression and become addicting. It's estimated that 10 percent of all cases of alcoholism begin when drinking is used as a way to deal with insomnia.[1]

Your sleep will most likely improve if you avoid alcohol entirely, but if you still want to drink, limit yourself to one drink at least 2 hours before you go to bed.

Avoid Caffeine after Lunch

Caffeine ingestion is a well-known cause of insomnia, especially if it occurs in the late afternoon/evening hours. It works by increasing production of a brain chemical called *norepinephrine*, which makes you more alert, anxious, and irritable—not a good thing if you're trying to fall asleep. Caffeine is also a natural diuretic, increasing the number of bathroom trips you have to make in the middle of the night. Finally, it can help wash away some of your supply of B vitamins, magnesium, potassium, zinc, and vitamin C, which can lead to blood sugar instability, water retention, migraine headaches, and mood changes. To reduce insomnia and avoid other caffeine-related problems, stay away from caffeine, especially after lunchtime. It can take hours to get it out of your system. (See "Take Care with Caffeine" section, page 86, in Chapter 5.)

Eat Complex Carbohydrates before Bed

A bedtime snack of whole-grain bread, crackers, cereal (unsweetened), or other foods high in complex carbohydrates can increase production of serotonin in the brain, which increases levels of melatonin and encourages sleep. However, if you eat a food high in protein at the same time, serotonin production will be inhibited. Don't confuse complex carbohydrates with simple carbohydrates (sugar, honey, fructose, etc.), which can ultimately cause a drop in blood glucose.

Beware of Sleep-Disturbing Foods

You want your body to wind down and be ready to rest when you go to bed. So don't burden it with foods that require special handling while you're trying to sleep.

- Foods high in sugar or refined carbohydrates, such as white bread, pasta, and pastry, can raise your blood sugar levels, then send them crashing down, interrupting sleep.
- Heavy, fatty foods take a long time to digest, so if you eat them close to bedtime, your digestive system will have to work overtime.
- Spicy foods, beans, or other gas-producing foods can cause indigestion that keeps you awake.
- Liquids taken during the hour or two before bedtime can trigger middle-of-the-night wake-up calls.

Supplements and Phytochemicals

Melatonin

Known for its ability to promote sleep and ward off the symptoms of aging, melatonin is a natural hormone converted from serotonin in the brain. Decreased levels of melatonin have been found in insomniacs of all ages and both sexes and may be one of the reasons that their sleep patterns become disturbed. Many studies of melatonin's effect on insomnia have shown positive results:

- Elderly insomniacs with melatonin deficiencies were given either 1 or 2 mg of a fast-release or a sustained-release melatonin tablet, or a placebo. The study's authors concluded that giving melatonin to insomniacs with a deficiency of the hormone helped to bring on and maintain sleep.[2]

- A study published in the prestigious British medical journal *Lancet* described what happened when 12 seniors suffering from insomnia were given melatonin. All of them took 2 mg of melatonin per day for 3 weeks, then a placebo for another 3 weeks. After they had taken the melatonin, the volunteers' sleep efficiency (the number of hours they actually slept divided by the number of hours they spent in bed) was significantly improved.[3]

- Knowing that small amounts of melatonin taken at noon increased the amount of melatonin in the blood at night and helped people fall asleep, researchers sought to find out what would happen if small doses of the hormone were given at night. Volunteers were given either a small dose of melatonin (0.3 or 1 mg) or a placebo in the evening or at night. Both doses of the hormone helped the participants fall asleep faster and move into deeper sleep sooner than the placebo did.[4]

Caution: Melatonin is believed to be safe for healthy people when used in moderation, for short periods of time, for the right reasons, and under the guidance of a physician. But it is a hormone and can affect many parts of the body, so it must be used with caution.

- Potential side effects include depression, headache, drowsiness, dizziness, irritability, and reduced alertness.
- You should not drive or use machinery for about 5 hours after taking the hormone.

- Taking melatonin along with alcohol or other central nervous system depressants, sleeping medications, or herbs or supplements with sedative properties, such as catnip, hops, or skullcap, might increase their effects.
- Melatonin may interfere with drugs designed to suppress the immune system.

Recommendations: There is no standard dose of melatonin. Many studies have used a bedtime dose of between 1 and 3 mg.

Valerian (Valeriana officinalis)

Valerian, which is sometimes referred to as the "herbal Valium," has traditionally been used for soothing migraines, rheumatic pains, and insomnia. German health officials have approved it for use as a mild sedative and sleep aid, and numerous studies suggest that the herb does indeed help ease insomnia.

- In 2000, Swiss researchers gave a valerian-hop combination to 30 people suffering from mild to moderate insomnia. After taking 500 mg of valerian and 120 mg of hops every evening for 2 weeks, the patients found that both the ability to fall asleep and their sleep efficiency improved. There were no side effects.[5]
- In the same year, researchers from the University of Miami gave between 470 and 1410 mg of valerian to 20 people suffering from sleep disturbances. The participants were asked to rate the effect of the herb on their insomnia using a scale of 1 to 5, with 1 being "no effect" and 5 being "extremely helpful." By the end of

the second week, 15 of the 20 rated the valerian as either a 4 or a 5.[6]

- Both a single dose and 2 weeks' worth of multiple dosages of valerian were compared to a placebo in a double-blind, placebo-controlled, crossover study with 12 women and 4 men, average age 49. The single dose was not effective, but the 2-week-long valerian treatment led to improvement in the time required to fall asleep, as well as to an increase in REM. The researchers concluded that valerian had "positive effects on sleep structure." Side effects were minimal, with the placebo causing more than the valerian.[7]

Caution: Although valerian has GRAS (Generally Recognized As Safe) status in the United States when taken for short periods of time, in the proper dosage, and for the right reasons, valerian usage is not without side effects.

- Potential side effects include headache, uneasiness, excitability, drowsiness the following morning and (ironically) insomnia.
- Using valerian can be habit forming, and it may cause withdrawal symptoms when you stop taking it.
- Taking valerian along with drugs or herbs that have sedating effects (e.g., kava, St.-John's-wort, alcohol, sedative drugs) could heighten their effects.

Recommendation: While there is no standard dose of valerian, some studies have used 400–450 mg of valerian liquid extract taken before bedtime for as long as 2 weeks.

Exercise

Insomniacs are generally more sedentary than people who sleep well, a fact that's not too surprising once you understand the effects of physical exercise on body temperature. A good aerobic exercise session will pump up your body temperature significantly, but 2–4 hours later your temperature will drop even lower than before you exercised. And a nice drop in body temperature is exactly what you need to bring on sleep. Exercise performed 3–6 hours before bedtime brings about the best sleep-promoting effects.[8] But don't exercise less than 3 hours before you go to bed, since your elevated temperature can cause the opposite effect. (A hot bath can cause similar rises and falls in body temperature, although the rise and fall occurs more quickly, and it's probably not as effective at promoting sleep as exercise is. Relax in a very hot bath for half an hour about 2 hours before bedtime.)

Exercise also eases tension, lessens anxiety, lifts depression, and has a natural tranquilizing effect. One study of 43 adults age 60 or older with insomnia found that exercise increased sleep duration and quality, and shortened the time it took to fall asleep.[9] For best results, moderately strenuous exercise should be performed at least 3 days a week for at least 30 minutes a session.

Lifestyle Changes

Adopt a Regular Bedtime
Nothing disrupts sleep faster than sleeping late on the weekend. Your internal clock becomes reset, so your body expects to go to bed later as well. But come Sunday night, when you're hitting the pillow

at your regular hour, your body thinks it's still got a couple of hours left to stay awake. This is the origin of the "Sunday night insomnia" that hits millions of Americans every weekend. To avoid it, pick a bedtime and a getting up time and stick with them, no matter what day of the week it is.

Keep Your Cool!

Now that you know how important a drop in body temperature is to both falling asleep and maintaining sleep, do what you can to make your sleeping environment cool:

- Keep the thermostat at 60 degrees or lower.
- Use 100 percent cotton nightclothes and sheets, for maximum absorbance and "breathability." You'll perspire less, or at least notice it less.
- Avoid flannel sheets, too many blankets, electric blankets, synthetic nightwear, or anything else that holds the heat in.
- Avoid hot baths right before bedtime. Warm showers are preferable.
- Use a fan to keep air circulating.
- Keep a wet, cool washcloth near your bed to help you cool down if you wake up in the middle of a hot flash.

Stop Smoking

The nicotine in cigarettes affects the brain in much the same way as caffeine, producing faster brain waves, increasing breathing and heart rate, and promoting higher levels of stress hormones. All of these stimulating effects can last for hours after your last cigarette and can keep you from falling or staying asleep. Also, sleep quality is diminished by nicotine withdrawal (which can occur in just a few hours) and smoke-induced irritation of the respiratory system. Not surprisingly, insomnia is a major complaint of smokers.

Relax

If you're uptight, worried, anxious, or troubled, you're not going to sleep well. But calling up the relaxation response, a deliberate quieting of the body and mind, can help relax your muscles, reduce your heart and breathing rates, lower your stress hormone levels, and help you drift off to sleep. Yoga, meditation, progressive relaxation, and listening to soothing music are just a few of the ways you can leave the stresses of the day behind. (See "Relax" under "Lifestyle Changes" in Chapters 7 and 8, pages 143 and 169, respectively.)

Consider Cognitive-Behavioral Therapy

Of the many types of psychotherapy, two may be especially helpful for insomniacs: cognitive and behavioral. In the case of chronic insomnia, cognitive therapy will focus in part on identifying negative attitudes toward sleep that can make it more difficult to fall or stay asleep. The cognitive therapist will help you replace these negative thoughts about sleep with positive ones. The goal is to reduce your stress and frustration regarding sleep so that you can relax and sleep better.

Behavioral therapy, on the other hand, will focus on practical strategies for improving sleep. In addition, the behavioral therapist will work with you on relaxation strategies and stress management. Research shows that cognitive and behavioral therapy, either alone or in combination, can help you get a good night's sleep.

- Twenty patients were given cognitive and behavioral therapy for 6 weeks, complete with bedtime restrictions, progressive muscle relaxation, and cognitive counseling. As a result of the therapy, sleep efficiency increased, the amount of time required to go to sleep decreased, and total sleep time increased from an average of 298 minutes to 381.[10]
- From the prestigious *Journal of the American Medical Association* comes a study with 75 adults who had been suffering from sleep-maintenance insomnia for an average of 13.6 years. Participants were given either cognitive-behavioral therapy, progressive muscle relaxation training, or a placebo therapy. They were treated for 6 weeks, and followed for another 6 weeks. Those receiving the cognitive-behavioral treatment did the best, enjoying an average sleep time of over 6 hours per night and the very good sleep efficiency rating of 85 percent.[11]
- Researchers from Johns Hopkins University reviewed 21 different studies comparing behavioral therapy to drugs and concluded that behavioral therapy was as effective as medications for the short-term treatment of insomnia.[12]

One of the great things about cognitive-behavioral therapy is that there aren't any side effects and you don't run the risk of developing an addiction. If your sleep troubles are persistent, see a psychologist and ask about cognitive-behavioral therapy.

Rising Stars?

We've talked about several natural therapies for insomnia in this chapter, but there are many more.

Here are some approaches that may prove to be valuable when more research with human subjects is conducted.

Acupuncture

A part of the larger system of traditional Chinese medicine, acupuncture attempts to treat disease by balancing the body's flow of energy. Thin needles, heat, electricity, and manual stimulation are used to influence the body's energy at specific acupuncture points. Acupuncture has long been used to treat sleep disorders, and some studies suggest that it might indeed deliver as promised. For example:

- In 1999, German researchers tested the effects of acupuncture on 40 people who had difficulty falling or staying asleep. The volunteers were split into two groups: one received acupuncture, the other fake acupuncture treatments that acted as a placebo. The results of the study showed that acupuncture was effective in treating sleep disorders.[13]
- Just over 30 people suffering from long-standing sleep disorders were enrolled in a study looking at the effects of needle acupuncture, laser acupuncture and cognitive therapy. Both traditional needle acupuncture and laser acupuncture helped relieve the sleep difficulties.[14]

Kava (Piper methysticum)

Although I could find no studies showing that kava directly influences sleep, its anti-anxiety effects have been widely documented. (See section on kava, page 161, in Chapter 8.) If your insomnia is stress-related, taking 60–120 mg of a standardized kava extract containing 30 percent kavalactones may help you relax enough so that you can fall asleep.

Light Therapy

If you live in a sunny area, you can increase your serotonin production just by taking a daily 10-minute walk in the bright sunlight without your sunglasses or tinted contacts. (Don't look directly at the sun.) If sunshine is frequently absent in your part of the world, you can purchase a special light box that provides fluorescent full-spectrum light similar to that of the sun. All you have to do is sit in front of the light box for 15–45 minutes per day (usually before 10 a.m.), reading, eating, or doing whatever you like. (Don't look directly at the light.) Light therapy stimulates the production of serotonin while decreasing its conversion to melatonin (which you don't want in the morning). However, the more serotonin you manufacture, the more "raw material" will be available for conversion to melatonin when it's time to go to sleep.

Melatonin helps us maintain sleep throughout the night, and those who wake up in the middle of the night may do so because their melatonin levels recede too quickly. In this case, using the light box in the evening may be an effective way to reset the melatonin cycle so that it starts later and recedes later.

Natural Progesterone

Since I began this chapter by telling you about my trials and tribulations with insomnia, I felt I couldn't end it without telling you what's worked best for me. The elusive "sleep juice" that I felt I just wasn't making enough of turned out to be progesterone. Once I started using natural progesterone in transdermal cream form, I relaxed, fell asleep much faster, and stayed asleep longer. Many perimenopausal women do notice a better, more restful sleep when using progesterone, which is not surprising since insomnia is one symptom of estrogen dominance.[15] Progesterone also helps alleviate other problems that can cause sleeplessness, like anxiety, depression, and erratic blood sugar levels.[16] And progesterone supplementation has a side effect that's great for us insomniacs: sleepiness! A recent study from *The Journal of the North American Menopause Society* found that both synthetic and natural progesterone increased sleep efficiency, but that natural progesterone worked best.[17] If you feel like you've forgotten how to fall asleep, it may be because you're lacking this important hormone.

Afterword

It's One-Third of Your Life!

Back in the days when women were primarily considered "baby-making machines," menopause signaled the onset of old age. But we who are currently going through menopause still have *one-third of our lives left to live*, and we're certainly not ready to be sidelined.

To tell you the truth, I'm still approaching menopause with a mixture of elation and dread. But as I've worked on this book, it's become increasingly clear to me that we *do* have some control over our destinies. Menopause doesn't have to be the gateway to old age. If we pay attention to our diets, exercise regularly, take certain supplements, and, above all, keep on top of what's going on in our bodies through regular doctor visits, we can probably avoid most (if not all) of the things that rob us of youth and vitality. We really *don't* have to develop heart disease or osteoporosis at some point down the line. We really *can* do something about the things that diminish joy and self-confidence, like incontinence, hot flashes, vaginal dryness, and depression. And it's absolutely possible for us to make it to old age with our health and sanity intact. But it takes work, and that work has to begin now, before the big problems set in. We're a lot more savvy about our health than our mothers or grandmothers were, and if we just apply what we know, we may be able to escape their health problems . . . for good!

Notes

Chapter One

1. Lee JR. *What Your Doctor May Not Tell You About Menopause.* (New York: Warner Books, 1996), 90.

2. Hulley S, et al. Randomized trial of estrogen plus progestin for secondary prevention of coronary heart disease in postmenopausal women. Heart and Estrogen/Progestin Replacement Study (HERS) Research Group. *JAMA* 1998; 280(7):605–13.

3. The HRT dose consisted of 0.625 mg of conjugated equine estrogens plus 2.5 mg of medroxyprogesterone acetate.

4. Herrington DM, et al. Effects of estrogen replacement on the progression of coronary-artery atherosclerosis. *N Engl J Med* 2000;343(8):522–29.

5. Writing Group for the Women's Health Initiative Investigators. Risks and benefits of estrogen plus progestin in healthy postmenopausal women. Principal results from the Women's Health Initiative randomized controlled trial. *JAMA* 2002;288(3):321–33.

Chapter Three

1. Centers for Disease Control. National Center for Chronic Disease Prevention and Health Promotion: www.cdc.gov/nccdphp/cvd/aboutcardio.html.

2. 2001 Heart and Stroke Statistical Update. Dallas, TX: American Heart Association, 2000.

3. Kalin MF, Zumoff B. Sex hormones and coronary disease: a review of the clinical studies. *Steroids* 1990; 55:330–52.

4. American Heart Association. "Heart and Stroke, an A-Z Guide": www.americanheart.org/HeartandStrokeAZ Guide/women.html.

5. Sen Biswas M, et al. Are women worrying about heart disease? *Women's Health Issues* 2002;12(4):204–11.

6. The Writing Group for the PEPI Trial. Effects of estrogen or estrogen/progestin regimens on heart disease risk factors in postmenopausal women. The Postmenopausal Estrogen/Progestin Interventions (PEPI) Trial. *JAMA* 1995;273(3):199–208.

7. Hulley S, et al. Heart and Estrogen/progestin Replacement Study (HERS) Research Group. Randomized trial of estrogen plus progestin for secondary prevention of coronary heart disease in postmenopausal women. *JAMA* 1998;280(7):605–13.

8. Henderson BE, et al. Estrogen replacement therapy and protection from acute myocardial infarction. *Am J Obstet Gynecol* 1988;159:312–17.

9. Hulley S, et al. Heart and Estrogen/progestin Replacement Study (HERS) Research Group. Randomized trial of estrogen plus progestin for secondary prevention of coronary heart disease in postmenopausal women. *JAMA* 1998;280(7)605–13.

10. Herrington DM, et al. The estrogen replacement and atherosclerosis (ERA) study: study design and baseline

characteristics of the cohort. *Controlled Clinical Trials* 2000;21:257–85.

Chapter Four

1. Kannel WB, Neaton JD, Wentworth D, et al. Overall and coronary heart disease mortality rates in relation to major risk factors in 325,348 men screened for the MRFIT, Multiple Risk Factor Intervention Trial. *Am Heart J* 1986; 112(4):825–36.

2. Wisser R. Conference on the health effects of blood lipids: Optimal distributions for populations. Workshop Report: Laboratory Experimental Section. American Health Foundation. *Prev Med* 1979;8:715–32.

3. McCarron DA, Reusser ME. The power of food to improve multiple cardiovascular risk factors. *Curr Atheroscler Rep* 2000;2:482–86. Hatton DC, Metz JA, Kris-Etherton PM, et al. Healthier diets improve quality of life while reducing cardiovascular disease risk factors. *Dis Manage Clin Outcomes* 1998;1:106–13. Renaud S, de Lorgeril M, Delaye J, et al. Cretan Mediterranean diet for prevention of coronary heart disease. *Am J Clin Nutr* 1995;61:1360S–67S.

4. Anderson JW, Gustafson NJ. High-carbohydrate, high-fiber diet: Is it practical and effective in treating hyperlipidemia? *Postgrad Med* 1987;82(4):40–55.

5. Eds. of UC Berkeley Wellness Letter. *The New Wellness Encyclopedia.* (Boston: Houghton Mifflin Co., 1995), 50.

6. Kromhout D. Dietary fatty acids, serum cholesterol, and 25-year mortality from coronary heart disease: The Seven Countries Study. *Circulation* 1992;85:864.

7. Robbins RC. Flavones in citrus exhibit antiadhesive action on platelets. *Int J Vitam Nutr Res* 1988;58:418–21. Puliero G, et al. Ex vivo study of the inhibitory effects of Vaccinium myrillus (Bilberry) anthrocyanosides on human platelet aggregation. *Fitoterapia* 1989;60(1):69–75.

8. Houston, MC. The role of vascular biology, nutrition and nutraceuticals in the prevention and treatment of hypertension. *J Amer Nutraceutical Assoc* 2002;Suppl.(1):5–71.

9. Gaby AR. "Coenzyme Q10" in *Textbook of Natural Medicine.* Pizzorno JE, Muray MT, eds. 2nd ed. (New York: Churchill Livingston, 1999), 663.

10. Janaki Y, Sugiyama S, Ozawa T. Ratio of low-density lipoprotein cholesterol to ubiquinone as a coronary risk factor. Letter. *N Engl J Med* 1991; 324(11):814–15.

11. Kamikawa T, et al. Effects of coenzyme Q10 on exercise tolerance in chronic stable angina pectoris. *Am J Cardiol* 1985;56:247.

12. Kato T, et al. Reduction of blood viscosity by treatment with coenzyme Q10 in patients with ischemic heart disease. *Int J Clin Pharmacol Ther Toxicol* 1990;28(3):123–26.

13. Fox B. *Foods to Heal By.* (New York: St. Martin's, 1992), 155–56.

14. O'Brien J. The first world congress on the health significance of garlic and garlic constituents: *Trends in Food Science and Technology* December 1990:155–57.

15. Winter R. *A Consumer's Guide To Medicines In Food.* (New York: Crown, 1995), 133.

16. Ernst E, et al. Garlic and blood lipids. *Br Med J* 1985;291:139.

17. Roberts AJ, O'Brien ME, Subak-Sharpe G. *Nutraceuticals: The Complete Encyclopedia of Supplements, Herbs, Vitamins and Healing Foods.* (New York: The Berkley Publishing Group, 2001), 476–77.

18. Singh RB, et al. Hypolipidemic and antioxidant effects of Commiphora mukul as an adjunct to dietary therapy in patients with hypercholesterolemia. *Cardiovasc Drugs Ther* 1994;8(4)659–64.

19. Gugulipid.com. Described in "Gugulipid": www.gugulipid.com/health.htm. Viewed November 22, 2002.

20. Life Extension Foundation. Described in "Benefits of Gugulipid (Commiphora mukul)": www.lef.org/protocols/prtcl-032.shtml.

21. Brown L, et al. Cholesterol-lowering effects of dietary fiber: a meta-analysis. *Am J Clin Nutr* 1999;69(1):30–42. Romero AL, et al. Cookies enriched with psyllium or oat bran lower plasma LDL cholesterol in normal and hypercholesterolemic men from Northern Mexico. *J Am Coll Nutr* 1998;17(6):601–08. Marlett JA, et al. Mechanism of serum cholesterol reduction by oat bran. *Hepatology* 1994;20(6):1450–57. Poulter N, et al. Lipid profiles after the daily consumption of an oat-based cereal: a controlled crossover study. *Am J Clin Nutr* 1994;59(1)66–69. Wursch, P, Pi-Sunyer FX. The role of viscous soluble fiber in the metabolic control of diabetes. A review with special emphasis on cereals rich in beta-glucan. *Diabetes Care* 1997;20(110):1774–80. Van Horn L. Fiber, lipids, and coronary heart disease. A statement for healthcare professionals from the Nutrition Committee, American Heart Association. *Circulation* 1997;95(12):2701–04. Rimm EB, et al. Vegetable, fruit, and cereal fiber intake and risk of coronary heart disease among men. *JAMA* 1996;275(6):447–51. He J, et al. Oats and buckwheat intakes and cardiovascular disease risk factors in an ethnic minority of China. *Am J Clin Nutr* 1995;61(2):366–72. Khaw KT, Barrett-Connor E. Dietary fiber and reduced ischemic heart disease mortality rates in men and women: a 12-year prospective study. *Am J Epidemiol* 1987;126(6):1093–102. Kwiterovich PO. The role of fiber in the treatment of hypercholesterolemia in children and adolescents. *Pediatrics* 1995;96(5Pt2):1005–09.

22. Romero AL, et al. Cookies enriched with psyllium or oat bran lower plasma LDL cholesterol in normal and hypercholesterolemic men from Northern Mexico. *J Am Coll Nutr* 1998;17(6):601–08.

23. Winblad I, et al. Effect of oat bran supplemented diet on cholesterolaemia. *Scand J Pri Health Care* 1995; 13(2):118–21.

24. Gerhardt AL, Gallo NB. Full-fat rice bran and oat bran similarly reduce hypercholesterolemia in humans. *J Nutr* 1998;128:865–869.

25. Keenan JM, et al. Randomized, controlled, crossover trial of oat bran in hypercholesterolemic subjects. *Journal of Family Practice* 1991;33(6):600–608.

26. Seidelin K, Myrup B, Fischer-Hansen B. N-3 fatty acids in adipose tissue and coronary artery disease are inversely related. *Am J Clin Nutr* 1992;55(6):1117–19.

27. Hu FB, et al. Fish and omega-3 fatty acid intake and risk of coronary heart disease in women. *JAMA* 2002;287(14):1815–21.

28. Dromhout D. N-3 fatty acids and coronary heart disease. *BNF Nutr Bull* 1990;15:93–102.

29. Seidelin K, et al. N-3 fatty acids in adipose tissue and coronary artery disease are inversely related. *Am J Clin Nutr* 1992;55(6):1117–19.

30. Castano G, et al. Effects of policosanol on postmenopausal women with type II hypercholesterolemia. *Gynecol Endocrinol* 2000;14(3):187–95.

31. Prat H, et al. Comparative effects of policosanol and two HNB-CoA reductase inhibitors on type II hypercholesterolemia. *Rev Med Chil* 1999;127(3):286–94.

32. Arruzazabala ML, et al. Effect of policosanol on platelet aggregation in type II hypercholesterolemic patients. *Int J Tissue React* 1998;20(4):119–24.

33. Arruzazabala ML, et al. Effect of policosanol successive dose increases on platelet aggregation in healthy volunteers. *Pharmacol Res* 1996;34(5–6):181–85.

34. De Lorimier AA. Alcohol, wine and health. *Am J Surg* 2000;180(5):357–61.

35. Waterhouse A, Frankel E, German JB, et al. The phenolic antioxidants in wine: Levels and effects. Paper presented

at the 208th American Chemical Society Meeting, Washington, D.C., August 22, 1994.

36. Corder R, et al. Endothelin-1 synthesis reduced by red wine. *Nature* 2001;414:863–64.

37. Coate D. Moderate drinking and coronary heart disease mortality: Evidence from NHANES I and the NHANES I follow-up. *Am J Publ Health* 1993;83:888–90.

38. Zhr Y, et al. Effects of Xuezhikang on blood lipids and lipoprotein concentrations of rabbits and quails with hyperlipidemia. *Chin J Parmacol* 1995;30:4–8.

39. Heber D, et al. Cholesterol-lowering effects of a proprietary Chinese red-yeast-rice dietary supplement. *Am J Clin Nutr* 1999;69(2):231–36.

40. Want J, et al. Clinical trial of extract of *Monascus purpures* (red yeast) in the treatment of hyperlipidemia. *Chin J Exp Ther Prep Chin Med* 1995;12:1–5.

41. Jenkins DJ, Kendall CW, Jackson CJ. Effects of high- and low-isoflavone soyfoods on blood lipids, oxidized LDL, homocysteine and blood pressure in hyperlipidemic men and women. *Am J Clin Nutr* 2002;76(2):365–72.

42. Anderson JW, et al. Meta-analysis of the effects of soy protein intake on serum lipids. *N Engl J Med* 1995;333(5):276–82.

43. Van Der Schouw YT, Pijpe A, Lebrun CE, et al. Higher than usual dietary intake of phytoestrogens is associated with lower aortic stiffness in postmenopausal women. *Arterioscler Thromb Vasc Biol* 2002;22(8):1245–47.

44. Roberts AJ, O'Brien ME, Subak-Sharpe G. *Nutraceuticals: The Complete Encyclopedia of Supplements, Herbs, Vitamins and Healing Foods.* (New York: The Berkley Publishing Group, 2001), 74.

45. Stensvold I, et al. Tea consumption. Relationship to cholesterol, blood pressure and coronary and total mortality. *Prev Med* 1992;21(4):546–53.

46. Green MS, Harari G. Association of serum lipoproteins and health-related habits with coffee and tea consumption in free-living subjects examined in the Israeli CORDIS study. *Prev Med* 1992;21:532–45.

47. Hertog MGL, et al. Dietary antioxidant flavonoids and risk of coronary heart disease: The Zutphen Elderly Study. *Lancet* 1993;342:1007–11.

48. Kono S, et al. Green tea consumption and serum lipid profiles: a cross-sectional study in northern Kyushu, Japan. *Prev Med* 1992;21:526–31.

49. Imai K, Nakachi K. Cross sectional study of effects of drinking green tea on cardiovascular and liver diseases. *Brit Med J* 1995;310:693–96.

50. Lou F, et al. A study on tea pigment in the prevention of atherosclerosis. Paper presented to the First International Symposium on the Physiological and Pharmacological Effects of *Camellia sinensis* (tea), New York, March 4–5, 1991.

51. Sato Y, et al. Possible contribution of green tea drinking habits to the prevention of stroke. *Tohoku J Exp Med* 1989; 157:337–43.

52. Morris DL, et al. Serum carotenoids and coronary heart disease—The Lipid Research Clinics Coronary Primary Prevention Trial and Follow-Up Study. *JAMA* 1994;272(18): 1439–41.

53. Gey KF, et al. Poor plasma status of carotene and vitamin C is associated with higher mortality from ischemic heart disease and stroke: Basel Prospective Study. *Clin Investig* 1993;71(1):3–6.

54. Gaziano JM, Hennekens CH. Antioxidant vitamins in the prevention of coronary artery disease. *Cont Int Med* 1995;7:9–14.

55. Gaby SK, Bendich A. "Vitamin B 12" in *Vitamin Intake and Health: A Scientific Review.* (New York: Marcel Dekker, 1991), 193–97.

56. Ibid. "Folic Acid," 175–83.

57. Dierkes J, Westphal S, Kunstmann S, et al. Vitamin supplementation can markedly reduce the homocysteine elevation induced by fenofibrate. *Atherosclerosis* 2001;158:161–64.

58. Kopjas TL. Effect of folic acid on collateral circulation in diffuse chronic arteriosclerosis. *J Am Geriatr Soc* 1966 14(11):1187–92.

59. Davis WH, et al. Monotherapy with magnesium increases abnormally low high density lipoprotein cholesterol: A clinical essay. *Curr Ther Res* 1984;36:341.

60. Mauskop A, Fox B. "New Hope From Nature" in *What Your Doctor May Not Tell You About Migraines.* (New York: Warner Books, 2001) 40–43.

61. Seelig MS. ISIS 4: Clinical controversy regarding magnesium infusion, thrombolytic therapy and acute myocardial infarction. *Nutrition Reviews* 1995;53:261.

62. Altura BM, Altura BT. Cardiovascular risk factors and magnesium: relationships to atherosclerosis, ischemic heart disease and hypertension. *Magnesium Trace Element: A Review* 1992;10(2-4):182–92.

63. Phillips P. Magnesium may extend survival after myocardial infarctions. *Medical Tribune* Sept 23, 1993;2.

64. Woods KL. Intravenous magnesium sulphate in suspected acute myocardial infarction. *Lancet* 1992:339 (8809):1553–8.

65. Gaby SK. "Niacin," in *Vitamin Intake and Health: A Scientific Review* (New York: Marcel Dekker, 1991), 189–91.

66. Guyton JR, et al. Extended-release niacin vs gemfibrozil for the treatment of low levels of high-density lipoprotein cholesterol. Niaspan-Gemfibrozil Study Group. *Arch Intern Med* 2000;160(8):1177–84.

67. Elam MB, et al. Effect of niacin on lipid and lipoprotein levels and glycemic control in patients with diabetes and peripheral arterial disease: the ADMIT study: A random-

ized trial. Arterial Disease Multiple Intervention Trial. *JAMA* 2000;284(10):1263–70.

68. Morato Hernandez ML, et al. Efficacy and safety of immediate-release niacin in patients with ischemic cardiopathy. Experience of the Instituto Nacional de Cardiologia "Ignacio Chavez." (Article in Spanish) *Arch Inst Cardiol Mex* 2000;70(4):367–76.

69. Roberts AJ, O'Brien ME, Subak-Sharpe G. *Nutraceuticals: The Complete Encyclopedia of Supplements, Herbs, Vitamins and Healing Foods*. (New York: The Berkley Publishing Group, 2001), 258–60.

70. Kok FJ, et al. Decreased selenium levels in acute myocardial infarction. *JAMA* 1989;261(8):1161–64. Virtamo J, et al. Serum selenium and the risk of coronary heart disease and stroke. *Am J Epidemiol* 1985;122:276.

71. Stead NW, et al. Selenium (Se) balance in the dependent elderly. *Am J Clin Nutr* 1984;39:677. Schiavon R, et al. Selenium enhances prostacyclin production by cultured epithelial cells: Possible explanation for increased bleeding times in volunteers taking selenium as a dietary supplement. *Thrombosis Res* 1984;34:389.

72. Korpela H, et al. Effect of selenium supplementation after acute myocardial infarction. *Res Commun Chem Pathol Pharmacol* 1989;65:249–52.

73. Roberts AJ, O'Brien ME, Subak-Sharpe G. *Nutraceuticals: The Complete Encyclopedia of Supplements, Herbs, Vitamins and Healing Foods*. (New York: The Berkley Publishing Group, 2001), 230–31.

74. Dierkes J, Westphal S, Kunstmann S, et al. Vitamin supplementation can markedly reduce the homocystine elevation induced by fenofibrate. *Atherosclerosis* 2001;158:161–64.

75. Rinehard JF, Greenberg LD. Vitamin B6 deficiency in the Rhesus monkey. *Am J Clin Nutr* 1956;4:318–25. Rinehard JF, Greenberg LD. Arteriosclerotic lesions in pyridoxine deficient monkeys. *Am J Pathol* 1949;25:481–96.

76. Dierkes J, Westphal S, Kunstmann S, et al. Vitamin supplementation can markedly reduce the homocysteine elevation induced by fenofibrate. *Atherosclerosis* 2001;158:161–64.

77. Krajcovicova-Kudlackova M, et al. Homocysteine levels in vegetarians versus omnivores. *Annals of Nutrition and Metabolism* 2000;44(3):135–38.

78. Khaw KT, Bingham S, Welch A, et al. Relation between plasma ascorbic acid and mortality in men and women in EPIC-Norfolk prospective study: a prospective population study. European Prospective Investigation into Cancer and Nutrition. *Lancet* 2001;357(9257):657–63.

79. Okamoto K. Vitamin C intake and apolipoproteins in a healthy elderly Japanese population. *Prev Med* 2002; 34(3):364–69.

80. Price KD, Price CSC, Reynold RD. Hyperglycemia-induced ascorbic acid deficiency promotes endothelial dysfunction and the development of atherosclerosis. *Atherosclerosis* 2001;158:1–12.

81. Boscobionik D, Szewczyk A, Azzi A. Alpha-tocopherol (vitamin E) regulates vascular smooth muscle cell proliferation and protein kinase C activity. *Arch Biochem* 1991; 286:264–70. Hennig B, et al. Protective effects of vitamin E in age-related endothelial cell injury. *Int J Vitam Nutr Res* 1989;59:273–79.

82. McQuilan, MB, et al. Antioxidant vitamins and the risk of carotid atherosclerosis. The Perth Carotid Ultrasound Disease Assessment Study (CUDAS). *J Am Coll Cardiol* 2001;38(7):1788–94.

83. Iannuzzi A, et al. Dietary and circulating antioxidant vitamins in relation to carotid plaques in middle-aged women. *Am J Clin Nutr* 2002;76(3):582–87.

84. Stampfer MJ, et al. Vitamin E consumption and the risk of coronary heart disease in women. *N Engl J Med* 1993;328(20):1444–49.

85. Kushi LH, et al. Dietary antioxidant vitamins and death

from coronary heart disease in postmenopausal women. *N Engl J Med* 1996;334(18):1156–62.

Chapter Five

1. American Heart Association. "High Blood Pressure Statistics": www.americanheart.org.

2. American Heart Association. "Women and Stroke": www.americanheart.org.

3. American Heart Association. "High Blood Pressure Statistics": www.americanheart.org.

4. Appel LJ, Moore TJ, Obarzanek E, et al. A clinical trial of the effects of dietary patterns on blood pressure. *N Engl J Med* 1997;336(16):1117–24.

5. Appel LJ. The role of diet in the prevention and treatment of hypertension. *Curr Atheroscler Rep* 2000;2:521–28. NHLBI. Clinical guidelines on the identification, evaluation, and treatment of overweight and obesity in adults—the evidence report. *J Obesity Res* 1998;6:51S–209S. Reisin E, et al. Effect of weight loss without salt restriction of the reduction of blood pressure in overweight hypertensive patients. *N Engl J Med* 1978;298(1):1–6. Conlin PR. Dietary modification and changes in blood pressure. *Curr Opin Nephrol Hypertens* 2001;10:359–63. Tuck ML, et al. The effect of weight reduction on blood pressure, plasma rennin activity, and aldosterone levels in obese patients. *N Engl J Med* 1981;304(16):930–33. McCarron DA, Reusser ME. Nonpharmalogic therapy in hypertension: from single components to overall dietary management. *Prog Cardiovassc Dis* 1999;41:451–60.

6. Appel LJ. The role of diet in the prevention and treatment of hypertension. *Curr Atheroscler Rep* 2000;2:521–28. Staessen J, et al. Body weight, sodium intake, and blood pressure. *J Hypertens* 1989;7:S19–23.

7. Houston M, Fox B, Taylor N. *What Your Doctor May*

Not Tell You About Hypertension. (New York: Warner Books, 2003), 117–19.

8. Joint National Committee on Prevention, Detection, Evaluation, and Treatment of High Blood Pressure. The sixth report of the joint national committee on the prevention, detection, evaluation, and treatment of high blood pressure. *Arch Intern Med* 1997;157:2413–46.

9. Hodgson JM, et al. Effects on blood pressure of drinking green and black tea. *J Hypertens* 1999;17:457–63. Sung BH, et al. Prolonged increases in blood pressure by a single oral dose of caffeine in mildly hypertensive men. *Am J Hypertens* 1994;7:755–58. Pincomb GA, et al. Acute blood pressure elevations with caffeine in men with borderline systemic hypertension. *Am J Cardiol* 1996;77:270–74. Cavalcante JW, et al. Influence of caffeine on blood pressure and platelet aggregation. *Arq Bras Cardiol* 2000;13:475–81.

10. Langsjoen P, et al. Treatment of essential hypertension with coenzyme Q10. *Mol Aspects Med* 1994;15:S265–S272.

11. Digiesi V, et al. Coenzyme Q10 in essential hypertension. *Mol Aspects Med* 1994;15:S257–S263.

12. Langsjoen P, et al. Treatment of essential hypertension with coenzyme Q10. *Mol Aspects Med* 1994;15:S265–S272.

13. Digiesi V, et al. Effect of coenzyme Q10 on essential hypertension. *Curr Ther Res* 1990;47:841–45.

14. Auer W, et al. Hypertension and hyperlipidaemia: garlic helps in mild cases. *Br J Clin Pract Suppl* 1990;69:3–6.

15. Steiner M, et al. A double-blind crossover study in moderately hypercholesterolemic men that compared the effect of aged garlic extract and placebo administration on blood lipids. *Am J Clin Nutr* 1996;64(6):866–70.

16. Qidwai W, et al. Effect of dietary garlic (Allium sativum) on the blood pressure in humans—a pilot study. *J Pak Med Assoc* 2000;50(6):204–7.

17. Silagy CA, Neil HA. A meta-analysis of the effects of garlic on blood pressure. *J Hypertens* 1994;12(4):463–68.

18. See, for example, Lungershausen YK, et al. Reduction of blood pressure and plasma triglycerides by omega-3 fatty acids in treated hypertensives. *J Hypertens* 1994;12(9):1041–45. Appel JK, et al. Does supplementation of diet with "fish oil" reduce blood pressure? *Arch Intern Med* 1993;153:1429–38. Morris MC, et al. Does fish oil lower blood pressure? A meta-analysis of controlled trials. *Circulation* 1993;88(2):523–33.

19. Morris MC, et al. Does fish oil lower blood pressure? A meta-analysis of controlled trials. *Circulation* 1993;88(2):523–33.

20. Toft I, et al. Effects of n-3 polyunsaturated fatty acids on glucose homeostasis and blood pressure in essential hypertension. A randomized, controlled trial. *Ann Intern Med* 1995;123(12):911–18.

21. Bao DQ, et al. Effects of dietary fish and weight reduction on ambulatory blood pressure in overweight hypertensives. *Hypertension* 1998;32:710–17.

22. Houston MC. The role of vascular biology, nutrition and nutraceuticals in the prevention and treatment of hypertension. *J Amer Nutraceutical Asso* 2002;(Suppl. 1):5–71.

23. Hasler CM, et al. Functional foods and cardiovascular disease. *Curr Atheroscler Rep* 2002:467–75.

24. Pereira MA, Pins JJ. Dietary fiber and cardiovascular disease: experimental and epidemiologic advances. *Curr Atheroscler Rep* 2000;2:494–502.

25. Vuskan V, et al. Konjac-Mannan (Glucomannan) improves glycemia and other associated risk factors for coronary heart disease in type 2 diabetes. *Diabetes Care* 1999;22:913–19.

26. McCarron DA, Reusser ME. Nonpharmacologic therapy in hypertension: from single components to overall dietary management. *Prog Cardiovasc Dis* 1999;41:451–60.

27. McCarron DA, et al. Blood pressure and nutrient intake in the United States. *Science* 1984;224(4656):1392–98.

28. Appel LJ, et al. A clinical trial of the effects of dietary patterns on blood pressure. DASH Collaborative Research Group: *N Engl J Med* 1997;336(16):1117–24.

29. Witteman JC, et al. A prospective study of nutritional factors and hypertension among US women. *Circulation* 1989;80(5):1320–27.

30. Griffith LE, et al. The influence of dietary and non-dietary calcium supplementation on blood pressure; an updated meta-analysis of randomized controlled trials. *Am J Hypertens* 1999;12:84–92.

31. Evans G, Weaver C, Harrington D, et al. Association of magnesium deficiency with the blood pressure-lowering effects of calcium. *J Hypertens* 1990;8(4):327–37.

32. See, for example, Kesteloot H, Joossens JV. Relationship of dietary sodium, potassium, calcium, and magnesium with blood pressure; Belgian Interuniversity Research on Nutrition and Health. *Hypertension* 1988; 12:594–99.

33. Witteman JC, et al. Reduction of blood pressure with oral magnesium supplementation in women with mild to moderate hypertension. *Am J Clin Nutr* 1994;60(1):129–35.

34. Witteman JC, et al. A prospective study of nutritional factors and hypertension among US women. *Circulation* 1989;80(5):1320–27.

35. Warner MG. Complementary and alternative therapies for hypertension. *Complementary Health Practice Review* 2000;6:11–19.

36. Barri YM, Wingo CS. The effects of potassium depletion and supplementation on blood pressure: a clinical review. *Am J Med Sci* 1997;3:37–40.

37. Hu G, Tian H. A comparison of dietary and non-dietary factors of hypertension and normal blood pressure in a Chinese population. *J Hum Hypertens* 2001;15:487–93.

38. Warner MG. Complementary and alternative therapies for hypertension. *Complementary Health Practice Rev* 2000;6:11–19. Appel LJ. The role of diet in the prevention and treatment of hypertension. *Curr Atheroscler Rep* 2000;2:521–28. Whelton PK, He J. Potassium in preventing and treating high blood pressure. *Semin Nephrol* 1999;19:494–99. Siani A, et al. Increasing the dietary potassium intake reduces the need for antihypertensive medications. *Ann Intern Med* 1991;115:753–59.

39. Barri YM, Wingo CS. The effects of potassium depletion and supplementation on blood pressure; a clinical review. *Am J Med Sci* 1997;314(1):37–40. Gu D, et al. Effect of potassium supplementation on blood pressure in Chinese: a randomized, placebo-controlled trial. *J Hypertens* 2001;19(7):1325–31.

40. Gu D, et al. Effect of potassium supplementation on blood pressure in Chinese: a randomized, placebo-controlled trial. *J Hypertens* 2001;19(7):1325–31.

41. Hajjar IM, et al. Impact of diet and blood pressure and age-related changes in blood pressure in the US population: analysis of the NHANES III. *Arch Intern Med* 2001;161(4):589–93.

42. Houston MC. The role of vascular biology, nutrition and nutraceuticals in the prevention and treatment of hypertension. *J Amer Nutraceutical Asso* 2002;(suppl. 1):5–71.

43. Pierdomenico SD, Constantini F, Bucci A, et al. Low-density lipoprotein oxidation and vitamins E and C in sustained and white-coat hypertension. *Hypertension* 1998; 31:621–26.

44. Koh ET. Effect of Vitamin C on blood parameters of hypertensive subjects. *J Okla State Med Assoc* 1984;77:177–82.

45. Duffy SJ, et al. Treatment of hypertension with ascorbic acid. *Lancet* 1999;354:2048–49.

46. Hajjar IM, et al. A randomized, double-blind, con-

trolled trial of vitamin C in the management of hypertension and lipids. *Am J Ther* 2002;9(4):289–93.

47. Houston M, Fox B, Taylor N. *What Your Doctor May Not Tell You About Hypertension.* (New York: Warner Books, 2003):156.

48. US Department of Health and Human Services. Physical Activity and Health: A Report of the Surgeon General. Atlanta, GA: Centers for Disease Control and Prevention, National Center for Chronic Disease Prevention and Health Promotion; 1996.

49. Predel HG. An exercise program for the hypertensive patient. Leaving hypertension behind. (Article in German) *MMW Fortschr Med* 2002;114(19):34-7. US Department of Health and Human Services. Physical Activity and Health: A Report of the Surgeon General. Atlanta, GA: Centers for Disease Control and Prevention, National Center for Chronic Disease Prevention and Health Promotion, 1996.

50. Tsai JC, et al. Beneficial effect on blood pressure and lipid profile by programmed exercise training in Taiwanese patients with mild hypertension. *Clin Exp Hypertens* 2002;24(4):315–24.

51. Tsai JC, et al. Beneficial effects on blood pressure and lipid profile of programmed exercise training in subjects with white coat hypertension. *Am J Hypertens* 2002;15 (6):571–76.

52. Whelton SP, et al. Effect of aerobic exercise on blood pressure: a meta-analysis of randomized, controlled trials. *Ann Intern Med* 2002;136(7):493–503.

53. Pescatello LS, Fargo AE, Leach CN, Scherzer HH. Short-term effect of dynamic exercise on arterial blood pressure. *Circulation* 1991;83:1557–61.

54. Moreau KL, et al. Increasing daily walking lowers blood pressure in postmenopausal women. *Med Sci Sports Exerc* 2001;33(11):1825–31.

55. Garrison R, Somer E. ''Hypertension, Smoking and

Cholesterol: The Primary Risk Factors" in *The Nutrition Desk Reference* (New Canaan, CT: Keats Publishing, 1995) 340–42.

56. Fuchs FD, et al. Alcohol consumption and the incidence of hypertension: the atherosclerosis risk in communities study. *Hypertension* 2001;37:1242–50. World Hypertension League. Alcohol and hypertension: implications for management. *WHO Bull* 1991;69:377–82. Altura BM, et al. Ethanol promotes rapid depletion of intracellular free Mg in cerebral vascular smooth muscle cells: possible relation to alcohol-induced behavioral and stroke-like effects. *Alcohol* 1993;10:563–66. Zhang A, et al. Ethanol-induced contraction of cerebral arteries in diverse mammals and its mechanisms of action. *Eur J Pharmacol* 1993;248:229–36.

57. Joint National Committee on Prevention, Detection, Evaluation, and Treatment of High Blood Pressure. The sixth report of the joint national committee on the prevention, detection, evaluation, and treatment of high blood pressure. *Arch Intern Med* 1997;157:2413–46.

58. Fuchs FD, et al. Alcohol consumption and the incidence of hypertension: the atherosclerosis risk in communities study. *Hypertension* 2001;37:1242–50.

59. Shapiro D, et al. Striking a chord: moods, blood pressure, and heart rate in everyday life.. *Psychophysiology* 2001;38(2):197–204.

60. Shapiro D, et al. Daily mood states and ambulatory blood pressure. *Psychophysiology* 1997;34(4):399–405.

61. Stetter F, Kupper S. Autogenic training: a meta-analysis of clinical outcome studies. *Appl Psychophysiol Biofeedback.* 2002;27(1):45–98.

62. Shapiro D, et al. Reduction in drug requirements for hypertension by means of cognitive-behavioral intervention. *Am J Hypertens* 1997;10(1):9–17.

63. Webb MS, et al. A progressive relaxation intervention

in the worksite for African-American women. *J Nat'l Black Nurses Assoc* 2000;11(2):1–6.

64. Leuchtgens H. Crataegus Special Extract WS 1442 in NYHA II heart failure. A placebo controlled randomized double-blind study. (Article in German) *Fortschr Med* 1993;111:352–54. Schussler M, et al. Myocardial effects of flavonoids from Crataegus species. *Arzneimittelforschung* 1995;45:842–45.

65. Siani A, et al. Blood pressure and metabolic changes during dietary L-arginine supplementation in humans. *Am J Hypertens* 2000;13:547–51.

66. Cherif S, et al. A clinical trial of a titrated olea extract in the treatment of essential arterial hypertension. (Article in French) *J Pharm Belg* 1996;51:69–71.

67. Nestel P, et al. Isoflavones from red clover improve systemic arterial compliance but not plasma lipids in menopausal women. *J Clin Endocrinol Metab* 1999;84(3):895–98.

68. Fuhita T, et al. Effects of increased adrenomedullary activity and taurine in young patients with borderline hypertension. *Circulation* 1987;75:525–32.

69. Asgary S, et al. Antihypertensive and antihyperlipidemic effects of Achillea wilhelmsii. *Drugs Exp Clin Res* 2000;26:89–93.

Chapter Six

1. American Academy of Orthopaedic Surgeons Online Service Patient Education Brochures. "Osteoporosis": orthoinfo.aaos.org/brochure.

2. McBean L, Forgac T, Finn SC. Osteoporosis: Visions for care and prevention—a conference report. *J of Amer Diabetic Assoc* 1994;94:668–71.

3. National Osteoporosis Foundation. www.nof.org/osteoporosis/stats.htm.

4. Gaby AR. *Preventing and Reversing Osteoporosis.* (Rocklin, CA: Prima Publishing, 1994), 2.

5. American Academy of Orthopaedic Surgeons Online Service Patient Education Brochures. "Osteoporosis": orthoinfo.aaos.org/brochure.

6. Browner WS, et al. Non-trauma mortality in elderly women with low bone mineral density. Study of Osteoporotic Fractures Research Group. *Lancet* 1991;338:355–58.

7. Writing Group for the Women's Health Initiative Investigators. Risks and benefits of estrogen plus progestin in healthy postmenopausal women. Principal results from the Women's Health Initiative randomized controlled trial. *JAMA* 2002;288(3):321–33.

8. Jilka RL, Takahashi K, Munshi M, et al. Loss of estrogen upregulates osteoblastogenesis in the murine bone marrow. Evidence for autonomy from factors released during bone resorption. *J Clin Invest* 1998;101(9):1942–50.

9. Ettinger B, Grady D. The waning effect of postmenopausal estrogen on osteoporosis. *Obstet Gynecol* 1996;87:897–904.

10. Schoenbeck L, Gibson CA, Barss MB. "Chapter 7: Bone Health" in *Menopause: Bridging the Gap Between Natural and Conventional Medicine.* (New York: Twin Streams, 2002).

11. Alaimo K, et al. Dietary intake of vitamins, minerals, and fiber of persons ages 2 months and over in the United States. Third National Health and Nutrition Examination Survey, Phase 1, 1988–91. *Adv Data* 1994;14(258):1–28.

12. Anderson JJB. Calcium, phosphorus, and human bone development. *J Nutr* 1996;126:1153S.

13. Breslau NA, Brinkley L, Hill KD, et al. Relationship of animal protein-rich diet to kidney stone formation and calcium metabolism. *J Clin Endocrinol Metab* 1988;66:140–46.

14. Soy.com. "Soy and Osteoporosis Technical Report": www.soy.com.

15. Itoh R, Suyama Y, Oguma Y, et al. Dietary sodium, an independent determinant for urinary deoxypyridinoline in elderly women. A cross-sectional study on the effect of dietary factors on deoxypyridinoline excretion in 24-h urine specimens from 763 free-living healthy Japanese. *Eur J Clin Nutr* 1999;53(11):866–90.

16. Nordin BE, Need AG, Steurer T, et al. Nutrition, osteoporosis and aging. *Annals of the New York Academy of Science* 1998;854:336–51.

17. Cummings SR, Nevitt MC, Browner WS, et al. Risk factors for hip fracture in white women. *N Engl J Med* 1995;332(12):767–73.

18. Hernandez-Avila M, et al. Caffeine, moderate alcohol intake and risk of fractures of the hip and forearm in middle-aged women. *Am J Clin Nutr* 1991;54:157–63.

19. Heaney RP, Recker RR. Effects of nitrogen, phosphorus and caffeine on calcium balance in women. *J Lab Clin Med* 1982;99:46–55.

20. Feskanich D, Singh V, Willett WC, et al. Vitamin A intake and hip fractures among postmenopausal women. *JAMA* 2002;287(1):47–54.

21. Courtesy of the Osteoporosis Program, Rhode Island Department of Health, 2002.

22. Horiuchi T, et al. Effect of soy protein on bone metabolism in postmenopausal Japanese women. *Osteoporosis International* 2000:11(8):721–24.

23. Scheiber MD, Rebar RW. Isoflavones and postmenopausal bone health: a viable alternative to estrogen therapy? *Menopause* 1999;6:233–41.

24. Hudson T. *Women's Encyclopedia of Natural Medicine.* (Los Angeles: Keats Publishing, 1999), 146.

25. Arjmandi BH, Birnbaum R, Goyal NV, et al. Bone-sparing effect of soy protein in ovarian hormone-deficient

rats is related to its isoflavone content. *Am J Clin Nutr* 1998;68:1364S–1368S.

26. Mei J, et al. High dietary phytoestrogen intake is associated with higher bone mineral density in postmenopausal but not premenopausal women. *J Clin Endocrinol Metab* 2001;86(11):5217–21.

27. Brynin R. Soy and its isoflavones: A review of their effects on bone density. *Alternative Medicine Review* 2002;7(4):317–27.

28. Alekel DL, et al. Isoflavone-rich soy protein isolate attenuates bone loss in the lumbar spine of premenopausal women. *Am J Clin Nutr* 2000;72(3):844–52.

29. Sugimoto E, Yamaguchi M. Stimulatory effect of daidzein in osteoblastic MC3T3-E1 cells. *Biochem Pharmacol* 2000;59(5):471–75.

30. Potter SM, et al. Soy protein and isoflavones; their effects on blood lipids and bone density in postmenopausal women. *Am J Clin Nutr* 1998;68(6 Suppl):1375S–1379S.

31. Ibid.

32. Heller HJ, Stewart A, Haynes S, et al. Pharmacokinetics of calcium absorption from two commercial calcium supplements. *J Clin Pharmacol* 1999;39(11):1151–54.

33. Cohen L, Kitzes R. Infrared spectroscopy and magnesium content of bone mineral in osteoporotic women. *Israeli J Med Sci* 1981;17:1123–25.

34. Angus RM, et al. Dietary intake and bone mineral density. *Bone Mineral* 1988;4(3):265–78.

35. Stendig-Lindberg G, et al. Trabecular bone density in a two year controlled trial of peroral magnesium in osteoporosis. *Magnes Res* 1993;6(2):155–63.

36. Cohen L, Kitzes R. Infrared spectroscopy and magnesium content of bone mineral in osteoporotic women. *Israeli J Med Sci* 1981;17:1123–25.

37. Rao DS. Perspective on assessment of vitamin D nutrition. *Journal of Clinical Densitometry* 1999;2(4):457–64.

38. Glerup H, Mikkelsen K, Poulsen L, et al. Commonly recommended daily intake of vitamin D is not sufficient if sunlight exposure is limited. *Journal of Internal Medicine* 2000;247(2):260–68.

39. Gaby, AR. "Vitamin K: As Important for Your Bones As Calcium" in *Preventing and Reversing Osteoporosis.* (Rocklin, CA: Prima Publishing, 1994), 21–28.

40. Knapen, MHJ, Hamulyak K, Vermeer C. The effect of vitamin K supplementation on circulating osteocalcin (bone GLA protein) and urinary calcium excretion. *Ann Intern Med* 1989;111:1001–5.

41. Hart, JP, et al. Electrochemical detection of depressed circulating levels of vitamin K1 in osteoporosis. *J Clin Endocrinol Metab* 1985;60:1268–69.

42. Tomita A. Postmenopausal osteoporosis Ca kinetic study with vitamin K2. *Clin Endocrinol* (Japan) 1971;19:731–36.

43. Knapen, MHJ, Hamulyak K, Vermeer C. The effect of vitamin K supplementation on circulating osteocalcin (bone GLA protein) and urinary calcium excretion. *Ann Intern Med* 1989;111:1001–5.

44. Feskanich D, Weber P, Willet WC, et al. Vitamin K intake and hip fractures in women: A prospective study. *Am J of Clin Nutr* 1999;69(1):74–79.

45. Knapen, MHJ, Hamulyak K, Vermeer C. The effect of vitamin K supplementation on circulating osteocalcin (bone GLA protein) and urinary calcium excretion. *Ann Intern Med* 1989;111:1001–5.

46. Ibid.

47. DeBenedette, V. Study: Swimming may increase bone density: *The Physician and Sportsmedicine* 1987;15(12):49.

48. Feskanich D, Willett W, Colditz G. Walking and

leisure-time activity and risk of hip fracture in postmenopausal women. *JAMA* 2002;288(18):2300–6.

49. Krall EA, Dawson-Hughes B. Smoking and bone loss among postmenopausal women. *Journal of Bone and Mineral Research* 1991;6(4):331–38.

50. Aloia JF, Vaswani AN, Yeh JK, et al. Determinants of bone mass in postmenopausal women. *Archives of Internal Medicine* 1983;143(9):1700–4.

51. Spencer H, et al. Alcohol-osteoporosis. *Am J Clin Nutr* 1985;41:847.

52. Prior JC. Progesterone as a bone-trophic hormone. *Endocrine Rev* 1990;11(2):386–98.

53. Prior JC, et al. Spinal bone loss and ovulatory disturbances. *N Engl J Med* 1990;323(18):1221–27.

54. Lee, JR. Osteoporosis reversal: the role of progesterone. *Int Clin Nutr Rev* 1991;10(3):384–91.

55. Reginster JY, et al. Trace elements and postmenopausal osteoporosis: a preliminary study of decreased serum manganese. *Med Sci Res* 1988;16:337–38.

56. Raloff J. Reasons for boning up on manganese. *Science News* 1986;130(Sept. 27):199.

57. Gaby, AR. "Boron" in *Preventing and Reversing Osteoporosis.* (Rocklin, CA: Prima Publishing, 1994), 59.

58. Nielsen, FH. Boron—an overlooked element of potential nutritional importance. *Nutr Today* 1988;(Jan./Feb.):4–7.

Chapter Seven

1. Schwingl PJ, Hulka BS, Harlow SD. Risk factors for menopausal hot flashes. *Obstetrics and Gynecology* 1994;84(1):29–34.

2. Berkow R, Beers MH, Fletcher AJ, eds. *The Merck Manual*

of Medical Information. (NJ: Whitehouse Station, Merck Research Laboratories, 1997), 1078.

3. Ibid.

4. Ivarsson T, Spetz AC, Hammar M. Physical exercise and vasomotor symptoms in postmenopausal women. *Maturitas* 1998;29(2):139–46.

5. Gannon L, Hansel S, Goodwin J. Correlates of menopausal hot flashes. *Journal of Behavioral Med* 1987; 10(3):277–85.

6. Staropoli CA, et al. Predictors of menopausal hot flashes. *J Womens Health* 1998;7(9):1149–55.

7. Ibid.

8. "Natural Menopause." The Gynecological Sourcebook, 3rd Edition. WebMD Health, webmd.com. http://my.webmd.com/content/article/1680.51664. Viewed December 10, 2002.

9. WebMD Health. Davis J. "Hot Flashes: Cursed Forever?" my.webmd.com/content/article/1689.54382. Viewed December 10, 2002.

10. Cameron M. "Menopause" in *Lifetime Encyclopedia of Natural Remedies.* (West Nyack, NY: Parker Publishing, 1993), 94.

11. Schwingl PJ, Hulka BS, Harlow SD. Risk factors for menopausal hot flashes. *Obstetrics and Gynecology* 1994;84(1):29–34.

12. Murray M. "Menopause" in *Encyclopedia of Nutritional Supplements.* (Rocklin, CA: Prima Publishing, 1996), 471.

13. Duker EM, Kopanski L, Jarry H, et al. Effects of extracts from Cimicifuga racemosa on gonadotropin release in menopausal women and ovariectomized rats. *Planta Med* 1991;57(5):420–24.

14. Einer-Jensen N, Zhao J, Andersen KP, et al. Cimicifuga

and Melbrosia lack estrogenic effects in mice and rats. *Maturitas* 1996;25(2):149–53.

15. Bodinet C, Freudenstein F. Influence of Cimicifuga racemosa on the proliferation of estrogen receptor-positive human breast cancer cells. *Breast Cancer Res Treat* 2002; 76(1):1–10.

16. Stolze H. An alternative to treat menopausal complaints. *Gynecology* 1982;3:14–16.

17. Lehmann-Willenbrock E, Riedel HH. Clinical and endocrinologic studies of the treatment of ovarian insufficiency manifestations following hysterectomy with intact adnexa. *Zentralblatt Fur Gynakologie* 1988;110(10):611–18.

18. Stoll W. Phytopharmacon influences atrophic vaginal epithelium: double-blind study: Cimicifuga vs estrogenic substances. *Therapeutikon* 1987;1(23)31.

19. Leiberman S. A review of the effectiveness of Cimicifuga racemosa (black cohosh) for the symptoms of menopause. *J Womens Health* 1998;7(5):525–29.

20. Liske E, Wustenberg P. Therapy of climacteric complaints with Cimicifuga racemosa: herbal medicine with clinical proven evidence. *Menopause* 1998;5:250.

21. Lock, M. *Encounters with Aging: Mythologies of Menopause in Japan and North America.* (Berkeley and Los Angeles: University of California Press, 1993.)

22. Adlercreutz H, et al. Dietary phyto-oestrogens and the menopause in Japan. *Lancet* 1992;339(8803):1233.

23. Messina M, Barnes S. The roles of soy products in reducing risk of cancer. *J Natl Cancer Inst* 1991;83:541–46.

24. ACOG News Release, January 31, 2000. "It's 'Buyer Beware' with Alternative Botanical Treatments for Menopausal Symptoms, Says ACOG": www.acog.org/from_home/publications/press_releases/nr05-31-01.cfm. Viewed December 12, 2002.

25. Murkies AL, et al. Dietary flour supplementation de-

creases post-menopausal hot flashes: effect of soy and wheat. *Maturitas* 1995;21(3):189–95.

26. Faure ED, et al. Effects of a standardized soy extract on hot flushes: a multicenter, double-blind, randomized, placebo-controlled study. *Menopause* 2002;9:329–34.

27. Nagata C, et al. Hot flushes and other menopausal symptoms in relation to soy product intake in Japanese women. *Climacteric* 1999;2(1):6–12.

28. Ivarsson T, et al. Physical exercise and vasomotor symptoms in postmenopausal women. *Maturitas* 1998;29(2):139–46.

29. Hammar M, Berg G, Lindgren R. Does physical exercise influence the frequency of postmenopausal hot flushes? *Acta Obstetricia et Gynecologica Scandinavica* 1990;69(5): 409–12.

30. Wallace JP, Lovell S, Telano C. Changes in menstrual function, climacteric syndrome and serum concentrations of sex hormones in pre- and post-menopausal women following a moderate intensity conditioning program. *Med Sci Sports Exerc* 1982;14:154.

31. Staropoli CA, et al. Predictors of menopausal hot flashes. *J Womens Health* 1998;7(9):1149–55.

32. Chiechi LM, et al. Climacteric syndrome and body-weight. *Clin Exp Obstet Gynecol* 1997;24(3):163–66.

33. Block A. Self-awareness during the menopause. *Maturitas* 2002;41(1):61–68.

34. Irvin JH, et al. The effects of relaxation response training on menopausal symptoms. *J Psychosom Obstet Gynaecol* 1996;17(4):202–7. Reynolds F. Some relationships between perceived control and women's reported coping strategies for menopausal hot flashes. *Maturitas* 1999;32(1):25–32.

35. Wijma K, et al. Treatment of menopausal symptoms with applied relaxation: pilot study. *J Behav Ther Exp Psychiatry* 1997;28(4):251–61.

36. Berkow R, Beers MH, Fletcher AJ, eds. "Menopause"

in *The Merck Manual of Medical Information*. (Whitehouse Station, NJ: Merck Research Laboratories, 1997), 1080.

37. Lee JR. "How to Use Progesterone Supplementation" in *What Your Doctor May Not Tell You About Menopause*. (New York: Warner Books, 1996), 276.

38. Loprinzi CL, et al. Megestrol acetate for the prevention of hot flashes. *N Engl J Med* 1994;331:347–52. Lobo RA, et al. DMPA compared with conjugated oesterogens for the treatment of postmenopausal women. *Obstet Gynecol* 1984;63:1–5. Aslaksen K, et al. Effect of oral MPA on menopausal symptoms on patients with endometrial carcinoma. *Acta Obstet Gynecol Scand* 1982;6:423–28. Schiff I, et al. Oral MPA in the treatment of postmenopausal symptoms. *JAMA* 1980;244:1443–45. Bullock JL, et al. Use of MPA to prevent menopausal symptoms. *Obstet Gynecol* 1975;46:165–68.

39. Leonetti HB, Longo S, Anasti JN. Transdermal progesterone cream for vasomotor symptoms and postmenopausal bone loss. *Obstet Gynecol* 1999;94:225–28.

40. Lee, JR. *What Your Doctor May Not Tell You About Premenopause.* (New York: Warner Books, 1999), 320–35.

41. Christy CJ. Vitamin E in menopause. *Am J of Obstet and Gynecol* 1945:50;84–87.

42. Smith CJ. Non-hormonal control of vaso-motor flushing in menopausal patients. *Chic Med* March 7, 1964.

43. Zava DT, Dollaum CM, Blen M. Estrogen and progestin bioactivity of foods, herbs and spices. *Proceedings of the Society for Exper Biol and Med* 1998;217(3):369–78.

Chapter Eight

1. Bruno, FJ. "Anger: Seeing Red When the Light Is Green" in *Psychological Symptoms* (New York: John Wiley & Sons, 1993), 23–29.

2. Cheraskin E, Ringdorf WM. *Psychodietetics: Food As Key to Emotional Health* (New York: Bantam Books, 1981), 72.

3. Yaryura-Tobias JA, et al. Phenylalanine for endogenous depression. *J Orthomolecular Psych* 1974;3(2):80–81.

4. Fisher E, et al. Therapy of depression by phenylalanine. *Arzneim Forsch* 1975;251:132.

5. Heller B. Pharmacological and clinical effects of DL-phenylalanine in depression and Parkinson's disease. In *Modern Pharmacology-Toxicology, Noncatecholic Phenylethylamines,* Part I. AD Mosnaim and ME Wolfe, eds. (New York: Marcel Dekker, 1978), 397–417.

6. Agren H, et al. Low brain uptake of L-[11C]5-hydroxytroptophan in major depression: a positron emission tomography study on patients and healthy volunteers. *Acta Psychiatr Scand* 1991;83(6):449–55.

7. Moore P, Landolt HP, Seifritz E, et al. Clinical and physiological consequences of rapid tryptophan depletion. *Neuropsychopharmacology* 2002;23(6):601–22.

8. Angst J, et al. The treatment of depression with L-5-hydroxytryptophan versus imipramine. Results of two open and one double-blind study. *Arch Psychiatr Nervenkr* 1977;224(2):175–86.

9. Zmilacher K, et al. L-5-hydroxytryptophan alone and in combination with a peripheral decarboxylase inhibitor in the treatment of depression. *Neuropsychobiology* 1988;20(1):28–35.

10. Shaw K, et al. Tryptophan and 5-hydroxytryptophan for depression. *Cochrane Database Syst Rev* 2002;(1):CD003198.

11. Volz HP, Kieser M. Kava-kava extract WS1490 versus placebo in anxiety disorders—a randomized placebo-controlled 25-week outpatient trial. *Pharmacpsychiatry* 1997;30:1–5.

12. Lehman E, et al. Efficacy of a special kava extract (Piper methysticum) in patients with states of anxiety, tension, and excitedness of nonmental origin—a double-blind

placebo-controlled study of four weeks treatment. *Phytomedicine* 1996;2:113–19.

13. Lindenberg D, Pitule-Schodel H. D,L-Kavain in comparison with oxazepam in anxiety disorders: a double-blind study of clinical effectiveness. *Fortschr Med* 1990;108:49–54.

14. Ernst E. The risk-benefit profile of commonly used herbal therapies: ginkgo, St. John's wort, ginseng, echinacea, saw palmetto, and kava. *Ann Intern Med* 2002; 136(1):42–53.

15. Greenwood CE, McGee CD, Dyer JR. Influence of dietary fat on brain membrane phospholipid fatty acid composition and neuronal function in mature rats. *Nutrition* 1989;5:278–81.

16. Stoll AL, Severus WE, Freeman MP, et al. Omega 3 fatty acids in bipolar disorder: a preliminary double-blind, placebo-controlled trial. *Arch Gen Psychiatry* 1999;56(5):407–12.

17. Hamazaki T, Sawazaki S, Itomura, M, et al. The effect of docosahexaenoic acid on aggression in young adults. A placebo-controlled double-blind study. *J Clin Invest* 1996;97(4):1129–33.

18. Woelk H. Comparison of St. John's wort and imipramine for treating depression: randomized controlled trial. *Brit Med J* 2000;321:536–39.

19. Philipp M, et al. Hypericum extract versus imipramine or placebo in patients with moderate depression: randomized multicentre study of treatment for eight weeks. *Brit Med J* 1999;319:1534–39.

20. Linde K, et al. St. John's wort for depression: an overview and meta-analysis of randomized clinical trials. *Brit Med J* 1996;313:253–58.

21. Bressa Gm. S-adenosyl-L-methionine (SAMe) as antidepressant: meta-analysis of clinical studies. *Acta Neurol Scand* 1994;89:7–14.

22. Young SN, Ghardirian AM. Folic acid and psychopa-

thology. *Prog Neuropsychopharmacol Biol Psychiatry* 1989;13:841–63.

23. Delle Chiaie R, et al. Efficacy and tolerability of oral and intramuscular S-adenosyl-L-methionine 1,4-butanedisulfonate (SAMe) in the treatment of major depression: comparison with imipramine in 2 multicenter studies. *Am J Clin Nutr* 2002;76(5):1172S–1176S.

24. Pancheri P, et al. A double-blind, randomized parallel-group, efficacy and safety study of intramuscular S-adenosyl-L-methionine 1,4-butanedisulphonate (SAMe) versus imipramine in patients with major depressive disorder. *Int J Neuropsychopharmacol* 2002;5(4):287–94.

25. Kagan BL, et al. Oral S-adenosylmethionine in depression: A randomized, double-blind, placebo-controlled trial. *Am J Psychiatry* 1990;147(5):591–95.

26. Mischoulon D, Fava M. Role of S-adenosyl-L-methionine in the treatment of depression: a review of the evidence. *Am J Clin Nutr* 2002;76(5 Suppl):1158S–61S.

27. Brozek J. Psychologic effects of thaimine restriction and deprivation in normal young men. *Am J Clin Nutr* 1957;5(2):109–20.

28. Benton D, Donohoe RT. The effects of nutrients on mood. *Public Health Nutr* 1999;2(3A):403–9.

29. Wyatt KM, et al. Efficacy of vitamin B6 in the treatment of premenstrual syndrome: systematic review. *Brit Med J* 1999;318(7195):1375–81.

30. Fafouti M, Paparrigopoulos T, Liappas J, et al. Mood disorder with mixed features due to vitamin B(12) and folate deficiency. *Gen Hosp Psychiatry* 2002;24(2);106–9.

31.Young SN, Ghadirian AM. Folic acid and psychopathology. *Prog Neuropsychopharmacol Biol Psychiatry* 1989;13:841–63.

32. Ibid.

33. Godfrey PS, Toon BK, Carney MW, et al. Enhancement

of recovery from psychiatric illness by methylfolate. *Lancet* 1990;336(8712):392–95.

34. Kaymar A. Elevation of mood with calcium and vitamin D. Paper presented at the 95th Annual Meeting of the American Psychological Association, New York City, August 31, 1987.

35. Thys-Jacobs S. Micronutrients and the premenstrual syndrome: the case for calcium. *J Am Coll Nutr* 2000;19(2):220–27.

36. Penland JG, Johnson PE. Dietary calcium and manganese effects on menstrual cycle symptoms. *Am J Obstet Gynecol* 1993;168(5):1417–23.

37. Dennerstein L, Dudley E, Guthrie J. Life satisfaction, symptoms, and the menopausal transition. *Medscape Womens Health* 2000;5(4):E4.

38. Dua J, Hargreaves L. Effect of aerobic exercise on negative affect, positive affect, stress and depression. *Percept Mot Skills* 1992;75(2):355–61.

39. Slaven L, Lee C. Mood and symptom reporting among middle-aged women: the relationship between menopausal status, hormone replacement therapy and exercise participation. *Health Psychol* 1997;16(3):203–8.

40. Kabat-Zinn J, et al. Effectiveness of a meditation-based stress reduction program in the treatment of anxiety disorders. *Am J Psychiatry* 1992;149(7):936–43.

41. Irvin JH, Domar AD, Clark C, et al. The effects of relaxation response training on menopausal symptoms. *J Psychosom Obstet Gynaecol* 1996;17(4):202–7.

42. Lee JR. *What Your Doctor May Not Tell You About Premenopause.* (New York: Warner Books, 1999), 64–65.

43. Ibid., 74–75.

Chapter Nine

1. LeBlanc ES, et al. Use of HRT may improve cognitive function in certain patients. *JAMA* 2001;284:1475–81, 1489–99.

2. Grady D, Yaffe K, Kristof K, et al. Effect of postmenopausal hormone therapy on cognitive function: the Heart and Estrogen/progestin Replacement Study. *Am J Med* 2002;113(7):543–48.

3. Seshadri S, Zornberg GL, Derby LE, et al. Postmenopausal estrogen replacement therapy and the risk of Alzheimer's disease. *Arch Neurol* 2001;58(3):435–50.

4. Mulnard RA, Cotman CW, Kawas C, et al. Estrogen replacement therapy for treatment of mild to moderate Alzheimer's disease: A randomized controlled trial. *JAMA* 2000;283(8):1007–15.

5. Ortega RM, et al. Dietary intake and cognitive function in a group of elderly people. *Am J Clin Nutr* 1997;66:803–9.

6. Jama JW, Lawner LJ, et al. Dietary antioxidants and cognitive function in a population-based sample of older persons. The Rotterdam Study. *Am J Epidemiol* 1996;144:275–80.

7. Foy CJ, et al. Plasma chain-breaking antioxidants in Alzheimer's disease, vascular dementia and Parkinson's disease. *Q J Med* 1999;92:39–45.

8. Gale CR, et al. Cognitive impairment and mortality in a cohort of elderly people. *Brit Med J* 1996;312:608–11.

9. Perrig WJ, et al. The relation between antioxidants and memory performance in the old and very young. *J Am Geriatr Soc* 1997;45:718–24.

10. Morris MC, et al. Vitamin E and cognitive decline in older persons. *Arch Neurol* 2002;59(7):1125–32.

11. Morris MC, et al. Dietary intake of antioxidant nutrients and the risk of incidence of Alzheimer disease in a biracial community study. *JAMA* 2002;287(24):3230–37.

12. Morris JC, et al. Vitamin E and vitamin C supplement use and risk of incident Alzheimer disease. *Alzheimer Disease Assoc Disorders* 1998;12;121–26.

13. Sano M, et al. A controlled trial of selegiline, alpha-tocopherol, or both as a treatment for Alzheimer's disease. *N Engl J Med* 1997;336:1216–22.

14. Alzheimer's Association. Morris JC. "Fact Sheet: Vitamin E": www.alz.org/ResourceCenter/ByTopic/vitaminE.htm. Paper last reviewed by Alzheimer's Association on October 1, 2002. Viewed December 22, 2002.

15. American Psychiatric Association. "Practice guideline for the treatment of patients with Alzheimer's disease and other dementias of late life. Part IV. Development of a treatment plan": www.psych.org/clin_res/pg_dementia.cfm. Guidelines published May 1997. Viewed December 22, 2002.

16. Doody RS, et al. Practice parameter: management of dementia (an evidence-based review). Report of the Quality Standards Subcommittee of the American Academy of Neurology. *Neurology* 2001;56(9):1154–66.

17. Engelhart MJ, Geerlings MI, Ruitenberg A, et al. Dietary intake of antioxidants and risk of Alzheimer disease. *JAMA* 2002;287(24):3223–29.

18. Cockle SM, et al. The effects of ginkgo biloba extract (LI 1370) supplementation on activities of daily living in free living older volunteers: a questionnaire survey. *Hum Psychopharmacol* 2000;15(4):227–35.

19. Mix JA, et al. A double-blind, placebo-controlled, randomized trial of ginkgo biloba extract EGb 761(R) in a sample of cognitively intact older adults: neuropsychological findings. *Hum Psychopharmacol* 2002;17(6):267–77.

20. Le Bars PL, et al. Influence of the severity of cognitive impairment on the effect of the ginkgo biloba extract EGb 761 in Alzheimer's disease. *Neuropsychobiology* 2002;45(1):19–26.

21. Le Bars PL, et al. A placebo-controlled, double-blind, ran-

domized trial of an extract of ginkgo biloba for dementia. North American EGb Study Group. *JAMA* 1997;278(16): 1327–32.

22. Le Bars PL, Kastelan J. Efficacy and safety of ginkgo biloba extract. *Public Health Nutr* 2000;3(4A):495–99.

23. Birks J, et al. Ginkgo biloba for cognitive impairment and dementia. The Cochrane Library, Issue 4, 2002. Oxford: Update Software Ltd.

24. Wilson RS, et al. Participation in cognitively stimulating activities and risk of incident Alzheimer's disease. *JAMA* 2002;287(6):742–8.

25. Seshadri S, et al. Plasma homocysteine as a risk factor for dementia and Alzheimer's disease. *N Engl J Med* 2002;346(7):476–83.

26. National Institutes of Health News Release. "High homocysteine levels may double risk of dementia, Alzheimer's disease, new report suggests": www.nih.gov/news/pr/feb2002/nia-13.htm. Viewed December 20, 2002.

27. Brooks JO 3rd, Yesavag JA, Carta A, et al. Acetyl L-carnitine slows decline in younger patients with Alzheimer's disease: A reanalysis of a double-blind, placebo-controlled study using the trilinear approach. *Int'l Psychogeriatrics* 1998;10(2):193–203.

28. Schreiber S, Kampf-Sherf O, Gorfine M, et al. An open trial of plant-source derived phosphatidylserine for treatment of age-related cognitive decline. *Isr J Psychiatry Relat Sci* 2000;37(4):302–7.

29. Roberts AJ, O'Brien ME, Subak-Sharpe G. *Nutraceuticals: The Complete Encyclopedia of Supplements, Herbs, Vitamins and Healing Foods.* (New York: The Berkley Publishing Group, 2001), 32–33.

30. Subhan Z, Hindmarch I. Psychopharmacological effects of vinpocetine in normal healthy volunteers. *Eur J Clin Pharmacol* 1985;28(5):567–71.

31. Allen JB, Gross AM, Aloia MS, et al. The effects of glucose on nonmemory cognitive functioning in the elderly. *Neuropsychologia* 1966;34(5);459–65.

32. Gold PE. Role of glucose in regulating the brain and cognition. *Am J Clin Nutr* 1995;61(4 suppl):987S-995S.

Chapter Ten

1. Leiblum S, Bachmann G, Kemmann E, et al. Vaginal atrophy in the postmenopausal woman. *JAMA* 1983; 249:2195.

2. Wilson, SK, Delk JR, Billups KL. Treating symptoms of female sexual dysfunction with the EROS-Clitoral Therapy Device. *J Gender Spec Med* 2001;4(2):54–58.

3. Handa VL, et al. Vaginal administration of low-dose conjugated estrogens: systemic absorption and effects on the endometrium. *Obstet Gynecol* 1994;84(2):215–18.

4. Smith, P. Estrogens and the urogenital tract: studies on steroid hormone receptors and a clinical study on a new estradiol-releasing vaginal ring. *Acta Obstet Gynecol Scand Suppl* 1993;157:1–26.

5 Messina M, Barnes S. The roles of soy products in reducing risk of cancer. *J Natl Cancer Inst* 1991;83:541–46.

6. Wilcox G, et al. Oestrogenic effects of plant foods in postmenopausal women. *Brit Med J* 1990;301:905–6.

Chapter Eleven

1. Heimer G, Samsioe G. Effects of vaginally delivered estrogens. *Acta Obstet Gynecol Scand Suppl* 1996;163:1–2.

2. Yoshikawa TT, et al. Management of complicated urinary tract infection in older patients. *J Am Geriatr Soc* 1996;44(10):1235–41.

3. Ibid.

4. Avorn J, et al. Reduction of bacteriuria and pyuria after ingestion of cranberry juice. *JAMA* 1994;271(10):751–54.

5. Kontiokari T, et al. Randomised trial of cranberry-lingonberry juice and *Lactobacillus* GG drink for the prevention of urinary tract infections in women. *Brit Med J* 2001;322:1571–73.

6. Smith P. Estrogens and the urogenital tract; studies on steroid hormone receptors and a clinical study on a new estradiol-releasing vaginal ring. *Acta Obstet Gynecol Scand Suppl* 1993;157:1–26.

7. Ishiko O, et al. Estriol, pelvic floor muscle exercises may combat post-menopausal stress incontinence. *J Reprod Med* 2001;46:213–20.

Chapter Twelve

1. Jacobs GD. *Say Good Night to Insomnia.* (New York: Henry Holt & Co., 1998), 120.

2. Haimov I, et al. Melatonin replacement therapy of elderly insomniacs. *Sleep* 1995;18(7):598–603.

3. Garfinkle D, et al. Improvement of sleep quality in elderly people by controlled-release melatonin. *Lancet* 1995;346(8974):541–44.

4. Zhdanova IV, et al. Sleep-inducing effects of low doses of melatonin ingested in the evening. *Clin Pharmacol Ther* 1995;57(5):552–58.

5. Fussel A, et al. Effect of a fixed valerian-hop extract combination (Ze 91019) on sleep polygraphy in patients with non-organic insomnia: a pilot study. *Eur J Med Res* 2000;5(9):385–90.

6. Dominguez RA, et al. Valerian as a hypnotic for Hispanic patients. *Cultur Divers Ethnic Minor Psychol* 2000;6(1):84–92.

7. Donath F, et al. Critical evaluation of the effect of vale-

rian extract on sleep structure and sleep quality. *Pharmacopsychiatry* 2000;33(2):47–53.

8. Jacobs GD. *Say Good Night to Insomnia.* (New York: Henry Holt & Co., 1998), 108.

9. Montgomery P, Dennis J. Physical exercise for sleep problems in adults aged 60+ (Cochrane Review). The Cochrane Library, Issue 4, 2002. Oxford: Update Software Ltd.

10. Backhaus J, et al. Long-term effectiveness of a short-term cognitive-behavioral group treatment for primary insomnia. *Eur Arch Psychiatry Clin Neurosci* 2001;251(1):35–41.

11. Edinger JD, et al. Cognitive behavioral therapy for treatment of chronic primary insomnia: a randomized controlled trial. *JAMA* 2001;285(14):1856–64.

12. Smith MT, et al. Comparative meta-analysis of pharmacotherapy and behavioral therapy for persistent insomnia. *Am J Psychiatry* 2002;159(1):5–11.

13. Montakab H. Acupuncture and insomnia. (Article in German) *Forsch Komplementarmed* 1999; Suppl 1:29–31.

14. Becker-Carus C, et al. Effectiveness of acupuncture and attitude-relaxation training in the treatment of primary sleep disorders. (Article in German) *Z Klin Psychol Psychopathol Psychother* 1985;33(2):161–72.

15. Lee JR. *What Your Doctor May Not Tell You About Premenopause.* (New York: Warner Books, 1999), 49–50.

16. Ibid., 60–62.

17. Montplaisir J, et al. Sleep in menopause: differential effects of two forms of hormone replacement therapy. *Journal of the North American Menopause Society* 2002;8(1):10–16.

Index

Nadine Taylor is chair of the Women's Health Council of the American Nutraceutical Association. She is the author of *25 Natural Ways to Relieve PMS* and *Green Tea: The Natural Secret to a Healthier Life,* as well as the coauthor of *What Your Doctor May Not Tell You About Hypertension, Arthritis for Dummies,* and *If You Think You Have an Eating Disorder.* A registered dietitian, she has lectured on health issues to various groups nationwide and written numerous articles on health and nutrition for the popular press.